THE DOCTOR IS BURNED OUT

THE

Doctor Is Burned Out

A Physician's Guide
to Recovery

JEFF MOODY, MD

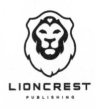

LIONCREST
PUBLISHING

THE DOCTOR IS BURNED OUT
A Physician's Guide to Recovery

ISBN   978-1-5445-0766-8 *Hardcover*
       978-1-5445-0765-1 *Paperback*
       978-1-5445-0764-4 *Ebook*

For Rachel, Sarah, Will, and always my Cheryl! For Kurt, who never burned out, and for Frankie and Simba, who got me up every morning to let them out and got me writing.

Contents

Author's Note: This is a deadly serious subject. Don't mistake levity on my part as insensitivity to the gravity of the situation. I am fighting to save the practice of medicine in the United States and the lives of my colleagues. For me, that includes the use of humor. But first, I had to save myself. Then my partners, friends, hospital, city, county, and state. I am ready. This book is an effort at "physician, heal thyself."

Throughout the book, I use the words *physician* or *doctor*. That descriptor can equally be applied or exchanged for "physician assistant," "nurse practitioner," "nurse," "veterinarian," other healthcare provider or anyone feeling lost, stuck, and burned out. All names and situations have been changed to protect privacy and patient confidentiality.

Introduction

I was surprised at how easily it broke in two. I had just emerged from my "frustration event" with the cracked halves of my keyboard, divided in the middle, with stray, homeless keys strewn across my desk.

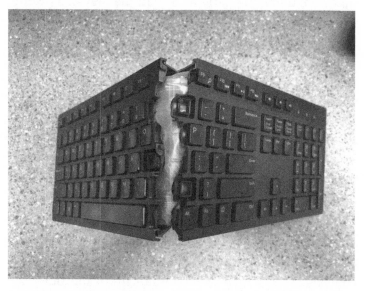

The death-of-a-thousand-cuts interaction I have with my electronic medical record (EMR), or as we affectionately refer to it as "that goddamn thing," usually involves endless clicking, freezes, and crashes. I had been pushed past my breaking point. Before I knew it, my keyboard was in pieces on my desk. I thought to myself, "Is this what my work life has become?" I know of physicians who have smashed computers, screens, or walls while expressing their frustrations with an EMR. The endless loop, failed integration, and helpless, hopeless time sink that had become the documentation of my patient visits had finally gotten the better of me. And to date, no randomized study has proven the utility of EMRs in improving healthcare or reducing costs.

In the previous year, I had two—count 'em two—reports filed at different hospitals for my behavior around frustration with expanding call coverage and hospital processes that were impeding patient care. In the previous twenty years? Zero. These seem to be symptoms of a larger problem: becoming burned out.

As physicians, we all walked fairly similar paths to get where we are. We were pleasers, achievers, doing things well, getting the prize/award/medal, and moving on to the next task. We were valedictorians, National Merit scholars, sports and debate champions, leads in school musicals. This process previously worked well; in fact, so well for me that I got a bonus present on my eighteenth birthday: I was diagnosed with a duodenal ulcer. I took cimetidine and was cured. Now stress instead causes me backaches or headaches. I took a brief hiatus from stress in my early college career, which yielded a fair bit of fun but very mediocre academic results. Gentle reminders from my parents about lack of parental support for lack of direction refocused me on my goals. I regained the academic high ground and was admitted to medical school.

This was probably the most important event in my life, not because I was now going to be a doctor but because this is where I met my future wife. She was at the next cadaver in Anatomy. It was very romantic, I know. They had a male cadaver. We had a female cadaver. We got to look at each other's parts—the cadavers', that is. My wife has single-handedly saved me at every point in my life. She encouraged me to "do whatever I need to be happy," including writing this book.

By the time of the keyboard event, I was definitely feeling burned out. I still love what I do, so what now? What next? How did I get so burned out? How do I fix this? Not my keyboard but my work-life balance, my pain points, and my burned-out results. My keyboard was beyond repair. Hopefully, my life and my career were not. I was trying to discern why I kept getting more and more frustrated every day, every week, every month with the demands on my time for things having nothing to do with patient care. I resented the theft of my energy away from me being the best I could be when I was with patients, friends, and family.

Are you frustrated, fatigued, fed up? Looking for answers or solutions? If this describes how you are feeling, this book is for you.

IN THIS BOOK, YOU WILL LEARN:
- What burnout is
- If you are burned out
- Why to change
- How to change

- What to change
- How to make systemic changes
- How to deal with change
- How to build a new, more satisfying, happy, productive life

YOU WILL NOT LEARN:
- How to accept your current situation
- Hopelessness
- Powerlessness
- That change is not possible
- That you are not worth the effort to change
- That you are alone

As a board-certified, UCLA-trained urologist with more than twenty years of experience, I thought that burnout was something that either was not supposed to happen to me or that I would have been trained to handle. That was not the case. Our training and experience make us great doctors but poor agents of self-diagnosis, care, and change.

One of my main motivations for writing this book was to show physicians and anyone else feeling burned out that you can indeed take back your power and hope. There can be dark times during burnout, where you might lose hope for improving your situation and your life. You may, like one of my friends, feel like suicide is your only option. I am fighting for your life. Seeing that you have power and hope are important aspects of burnout treatment. You will be opening your mind and perception to the idea that you are not boxed in, that you have a broad range of gifts and abilities, and can improve, create, and grow into a new, enhanced identity.

There are many options available to you and essentially an infinite number of paths open for you to follow. These paths may not be the ones you thought you would be taking one, five, or ten years ago. They may or may not include medicine as a component. Open your mind to the possibilities. Throughout this book, we will be bringing a new "you" into being.

Asking you to potentially change your current situation is a major step. I know you spent ten to fifteen years, through undergrad, medical school, and residency getting to the point where you can do what you thought you wanted to do. Your "switching costs," meaning the perceived or actual cost of changing what you do, are high. In business, and in medicine, those characteristics can be considered competitive advantages or "moats" preventing others from getting in and competing with you. However, from a burnout perspective, those moats may be keeping you inside. All I am asking is that you realize your life, moats and all, may be harming you.

As a doctor, who has been burned out, is now recovered, and taught others how to recover from burnout, I can help you get there. You are going through a process of bringing this new "you" into being. This can be a disorienting process, as you transition from the current "you" to the new one. Through this book, you will be learning, doing exercises of assessment, taking action, and directing your life, wherever you want to go. This is what I still do every day.

Let's start from where you are, define your path, and get you there: Recovered from Burnout.

PART I

The Burnout Crisis

CHAPTER 1

The Mental Health of Burnout

Why? Why Me? Why Now? Why This Book?

"If your why is strong enough, you will figure out how."

—BILL WALSH

You might ask yourself, "Why is this guy writing a book about burnout? Isn't he a successful doctor? What does he have to be burned out about?" Those are questions we will explore throughout the rest of the book. I had to go through the following process to diagnose, treat, and recover from burnout.

Let me tell you why this book is important to me. Every day in the United States, on average, one doctor kills him- or herself. The causes are varied and unknown. It may be a combination of stress, fatigue, anxiety, depression, hopelessness, entrapment, or futility. It could be the nonstop pressure to perform without errors. Or it simply may be a lack of knowing how to care for oneself and what options exist for the future. More than 50 percent of physicians are clinically burned out, 70 percent would not recommend medicine as a career, one in seven are suicidal, and one per day completes suicide.

I want this book to take the dark curtain off physicians in need of help and let them step into the light of healing. There is nothing like a little light and air on a problem to dispel the bad humors. Shining the light on myself, I hope, will encourage others to recognize their own issues, seek care, and no longer feel the stigma of seeking care for mental health issues.

My burnout was not severe enough that there were negative, long-term consequences. Colleagues have told me in retrospect that they had no idea I was burning out. I didn't show off my burnout—much—although those closest to me saw the anger and frustration. What I do know is the current state of mental health within the medical community is in crisis.

Let me turn that around on you: "Why are you reading this book?" My hunch is that if things were perfect, you would be scrolling through your favorite social media app, reading historical fiction, or improving your fly-fishing. Have you had second thoughts about reading this book for fear of someone seeing you reading a book about burnout? Ah, yes, you can't let anyone know you might be burned out. Let's explore the mental health aspects of life as a physician.

There is a giant stigma in medicine attached to physicians seeking care for mental health issues, trauma, and substance use and abuse. No physician likes to consider that they may need help to deal with the enormous stresses of the job. Physicians are all, of course, perfectly mentally healthy and never have issues that may need counseling, medicine, or changes in their lives. Or not! We have just as many issues as everybody else. We just are not supposed to have them.

No job, other than perhaps airline pilots, requires you to regularly answer questionnaires asking if you have any health issues, mental or physical, that would prevent you from performing your job like medicine does. At least airline pilots have a no-fault reporting system for any issues they may be having. I am required to answer these mental and physical health questions more than ten times per year, every time I fill out an application for privileges for a hospital, an insurance plan, or board certification. Below is an actual set of questions I had to complete for reapplication of my privileges at a local hospital while writing this book.

DISCLOSURE—COMPLETED BY ALL APPLICANTS AT INITIAL APPOINTMENT AND AT REAPPOINTMENT

Indicate yes or no for each question.

If the answer is yes to any of the following, please provide details on a separate sheet of paper.

1. Has your license to practice medicine or any other health profession and/or your federal or state registration or permit to prescribe narcotics or other drugs in any jurisdiction ever been voluntarily or involuntarily denied, restricted, suspended, revoked or not renewed, and any currently pending challenges thereof?

2. Have you ever voluntarily withdrawn an application, surrendered or not renewed your license to practice medicine or any other profession in any jurisdiction?

3. Have you ever been formally charged by, received a reprimand from or been placed on probation by a professional licensing or disciplinary authority in any jurisdiction?

4. To the best of your knowledge, are you currently, or within the last 5 years, have you been the subject of a complaint or investigation by a professional licensing/disciplinary agency, a peer review or quality assurance committee at a licensed facility or a professional or specialty society in any jurisdiction?

5. Have you ever been involuntarily terminated or been forced to resign from a clinical position with the armed forces or any federal, state or local agency, or any other professional employment or practice arrangement, or have you ever resigned voluntarily while under investigation or threat of sanction?

6. Have you ever voluntarily accepted sanctions or restrictions on your ability to practice under threat of same or voluntarily resigned under threat of same from any of those entities listed in the preceding question?

7. Have you ever been reprimanded, censured, or otherwise disciplined by a certifying, registering or licensing agency, a professional society, a medical staff, or a licensed facility?

8. Has your request for specific clinical privileges or medical staff membership with a licensed facility ever been denied or granted with stated limitation, or have any of your privileges been voluntarily or involuntarily suspended, revoked, resigned, surrendered, withdrawn or not renewed at a licensed facility?

9. Have you ever been denied membership in a professional or specialty society?

10. Have you ever been convicted of any felony or any misdemeanor involving drugs, alcohol, or in any way the practice of medicine or any other health profession or do you now have such charges pending against you?

11. Have you ever been subjected to civil or criminal penalties under the Medicare or Medicaid program?

12. Have you ever been suspended from participation in Medicare or Medicaid?

13. In the time since you began practicing medicine, have there been any gaps or periods that you were not practicing medicine?

14. Do you use any chemical substance that would in any way impair or limit your ability to practice medicine and perform the functions of your job with reasonable skill and safety?

15. Is there any reason you are unable to perform all the procedures for which you requested privileges, with or without accommodation, according to accepted standards of professional performance without posing a threat to patient, nursing staff, administrative staff or other medical staff?

16. Are you currently engaged in illegal use of any legal or illegal substances?

17. Do you have any physical, mental, or emotional condition that would affect your clinical performance and judgment in any way?

18. Are you currently under any limitations in terms of activity or workload?

19. Have you had a refusal or cancellation of professional liability coverage?

20. During the past four (4) years, have you been named in or the subject of any malpractice claims and/or suits?

Signature: _____   Date: _____

Print Name: _____

The concern for physicians is the fact that admitting to mental health issues or seeking help for those same issues could be construed as not being able to perform your job. So there is considerable pressure on physicians to perform and ignore any issues, lest they interfere with their job, their licensure, their privileges, their perceived competence, and their livelihood. Studies show that concerns by physicians about licensure loss and interventions hamper seeking mental health care.[1] A study of American surgeons showed 60 percent did not seek mental health care for suicidal ideation due to concerns over loss of licensure.[2]

I saw a therapist for several years while I dealt with some frustration issues. Because of my concerns about anyone knowing that I saw a therapist, I told no one. And, of course, I paid cash and did not run it through my health insurance. Outside of my family, this is the first time I have shared this with anyone. I guess that cat is out of the bag in a giant way. My therapist helped me work through my issues, and I consider him a friend and a great resource to whom I refer others needing his services. Qualified mental

1   K. J. Gold et al., "'I Would Never Want to Have a Mental Health Diagnosis on My Record': A Survey of Female Physicians on Mental Health Diagnosis, Treatment, and Reporting," *General Hospital Psychiatry* 43 (November–December 2016): 51–57.

2   T. D. Shanafelt et al., "Special Report: Suicidal Ideation among American Surgeons," *Archives of Surgery* 146, no. 1 (January 2011): 54–62.

health professionals, therapists, psychologists, and psychiatrists all stand ready to help. You just need to raise your hand for help, which can be difficult. I know! It is OK to be the patient for once and get the help you need.

Education around mental health is beneficial for physicians. To that end, I have recently completed my health systems' peer coaching program to identify and interact with physicians experiencing burnout.

PHYSICIAN HEALTH PROGRAMS

On the state level, there are organizations called Physician Health Programs (PHPs). These provide valuable resources and mechanisms for treating physicians with medical, substance abuse, or other issues that may impair their ability to practice medicine.

Most state PHPs govern and implement the treatment of impaired physicians referred or directed to them. The referral process to a state PHP can be anonymous but is typically done by a reporting person or agency or is mandated by legal action. In my state, the mandated referral rate of all the physicians treated is 40 percent.[3] PHPs coordinate treatment and monitoring for physicians, increase patient safety, and reduce malpractice.[4] [5] There are some physician concerns about oversight, transpar-

---

3   Colorado Physician Health Program, *2018 Annual Report*, p. 2.

4   Elizabeth Brooks, Doris C. Gundersen, and Michael H. Gundersen, "Investing in Physicians Is Investing in Patients: Enhancing Patient Safety through Physician Health and Well-Being Research," *MD Journal of Patient Safety*. doi: 10.1097/PTS.0000000000000318.

5   *Occupational Medicine* 63, no. 4 (June 1, 2013): 274–280.

ency, or mechanism of action by PHPs.[6] In fact, in a recent survey, only 6 percent of physicians have or would seek help through a PHP due to concerns for privacy, licensure action, or effects on their ability to practice medicine.[7] The PHP does work with but not under the oversight of state medical boards.

A number of states have adopted "safe haven" statutes, which allow a physician to answer no to questions about any health issues affecting their ability to practice medicine, once they have been treated by a PHP. This is a step in the right direction of destigmatizing the process of seeking and obtaining care.

If the process was more supportive and less punitive, many more physicians would step forward to get help. Are there doctors who have substance abuse or other issues that preclude them from giving appropriate care? Yes. PHPs exist to help those physicians. But the vast majority of physicians who could benefit from mental health care simply do not seek care due to concerns, real or imagined, about their perceived competence, restrictions on their license, and ultimately, their ability to practice medicine.

Doctors will ignore or refuse to acknowledge their own health issues in order to be able to work at a profession they spent ten to fifteen years training to do. There is significant pressure to perform as a physician, regardless of the mental health effects. At no time can weakness or infirmity be shown, at least as we are trained and reinforced to believe.

---

6   https://www.medschooltutors.com/blog/the-dark-side-of-physician-health-programs

7   *Medscape National Physician Burnout, Depression & Suicide Report 2019*, slide 21.

The appropriate way to encourage identification, care, and help for those physicians with non-substance abuse or mental health issues is less clear. A positive step would be a mechanism to make seeking care for mental health by physicians nonjudgmental, open, and stress relieving. Normalizing and discussing mental health care would open the door for healing for the healers. We will explore systemic solutions for physician mental health in chapter 20.

Would you not seek treatment for diabetes or high blood pressure? No! So why not treat burnout, dysthymia, depression, ADD, or insomnia due to stress? Substance abuse or addiction are also real diseases with real consequences no matter who you are. They deserve appropriate diagnosis, treatment, and ongoing care. Absolutely seek care whenever you need it! My why is clear to me. It led me to how. Let's define the problem of burnout, and get to your why and how!

CHAPTER 1 TAKEAWAYS

- Why here and now? Because it is time to change your life and start your recovery from burnout.
- Suicide can be a result of burnout.
- Mental health is a significant component of your life.
- Mental health needs to be brought into mainstream care for everyone, including physicians.
- PHPs help impaired physicians return to practice.
- A process for allowing physicians to access mental health care in an open, uncritical way is paramount to changing the future of burnout.

CHAPTER 2

Burnout Definitions

"You will burn and you will burn out; you will be healed and come back again."

—FYODOR DOSTOEVSKY

I hate to argue with a famous, dead Russian author, but I do not think burnout is inevitable from a medical career standpoint, but recovery is absolutely possible if burnout occurs. But first, in medicine, we want to define the problem. This helps us outline the scope of the problem, where we are, what the research says about appropriate therapy, and what our options are going forward. As a physician suffering from burnout, I wanted to know where I was and where I could go. Once we know the possibilities, then we pursue action. I tell my patients that life is full of choices, and we have the power to choose a course of action.

Let's define the problem, the drivers of burnout, the results of burnout, and see what the options are. We will fully explore our treatment options beginning in chapter 8. We need to examine how we got here, both personally and as a profession.

When it comes to burnout, there are different definitions of what that means. It is classically defined as a symptom constellation of emotional exhaustion, depersonalization, and diminished personal accomplishment at work.[8] Experts speak of burnout as emotional and ethical exhaustion due to stress. My personal dark horse favorite is the Urban Dictionary definition of burnout as "a state of emotional and physical exhaustion caused by a prolonged period of stress and frustration; an inevitable corporate condition characterized by frequent displays of unprofessional behavior, a blithe refusal to do any work, and most important, a distinct aura of not giving a shit."

One of my friends, a hospitalist from Texas, does not like or use the term *burnout*. He prefers to think of and label it as straight-up abuse of physicians, our abilities, and our sense of duty. I can't say I disagree. Others have spoken about what physicians endure as "moral injury" and even a "human rights violation." I really am not married to any particular term. What is happening is deadly serious, and we, as a profession, cannot continue to work and respond in the same way. We cannot allow the current system to continue without active change by us for us.

My own definition of burnout is this: The lack of value received by me for aligned effort that is simultaneously efficient, correct, and well done, which results in frustration, fatigue, anger, discontentment, and depression. As physicians, we give and give and give, creating value for our patients, our staff, and our hospitals. Yes, we are compensated for what we do. What is demanded by the healthcare system in exchange for that value is dispropor-

---

8   C. Maslach and S. E. Jackson, *Maslach Burnout Inventory* (Palo Alto, CA: Consulting Psychologists Press, 1986).

tionate. We spend hours saving a life but then are asked to spend more hours completing time-wasting tasks for the benefit of the rest of the system.

The value we create accrues not to us but to the hospital, insurance company, or other party. Numerous physicians I have spoken with relate that lack of being valued is a significant source of their burnout. These multifactorial demands on time, effort, compliance, work-life balance, mental and physical health, and life are endless and increasing. Compensation declines every year. This perfect storm of negative events increases burnout.

Burnout has been evaluated historically by the Maslach Burnout Inventory (MBI).[9] This is a series of questions designed to evaluate three axes of mental status: exhaustion/emotional overwhelm, depersonalization/cynicism, and lack of personal accomplishment. The inventory was initially designed to evaluate social workers and their state of mental exhaustion and burnout. However, the inventory has been validated for use with physicians as well.[10] It is a useful tool to know if and how much someone is burned out and to track treatment success over time.

Physician burnout is not just an American problem. There is a long history of varying degrees of burnout in physicians from other countries. Stress and burnout in colorectal and vascular surgical consultants working in the UK was studied in 2007. At that time, 32 percent of surgeons had high burnout on at least one subscale

---

9   *Maslach Burnout Inventory*, 3rd ed. (Palo Alto, CA: Consulting Psychologists Press, 1997).

10   J. P. Rafferty et al., "Validity of the Maslach Burnout Inventory for Family Practice Physicians," *Journal of Clinical Psychology* 42, no. 3 (1986): 488–492.

of the MBI, and 77 percent stated that they intended to retire before the statutory retirement age.[11] A large meta-analysis of 9,300 physicians in China yielded an overall prevalence of burnout symptoms ranging from 66 percent to 88 percent.[12]

However, not all countries report high burnout rates. In a study of rural Japanese physicians, only 22 percent had burnout and 10 percent of the doctors intended to resign. In further analysis, high ability to control job factors for these physicians had a significantly protective effect against burnout.[13]

However, physicians do not seem to be the only workers who are burning out. Burnout is rising in all workers in the United States. A survey found 27.8 percent of American workers had symptoms of burnout in 2011.[14] This had increased to 40 percent by 2016.[15] This leads to damaging effects on the working population. According to a Gallup survey, those same burned-out workers were 63 percent more likely to take a sick day, 23 percent more likely to visit an emergency room, and 2.6 times more likely to leave their current employer.[16] Burnout actually increases usage

11   *Psycho-Oncology* 17 (2008): 570–576.

12   D. Lo, F. Wu, M. Chan, and D. Li, "A Systematic Review of Burnout among Doctors in China: A Cultural Perspective," *Asia Pacific Family Medicine* 17(February 8, 2018): 3.

13   *Tohoku Journal of Experimental Medicine* 245 (2018): 167–177.

14   T. D. Shanafelt et al., "Burnout and Satisfaction with Work-Life Balance among US Physicians Relative to the General US Population," *Archive of Internal Medicine* 172, no. 18 (2012): 1377–1385.

15   Staples Business Advantage, *Workplace Index 2016* (Framingham, MA: Staples, 2016).

16   B. Wigert and S. Agrawal, *Employee Burnout, Part 1: The 5 Main Causes*, July 18, 2018, https://www.gallup.com/workplace/237059/employee-burnout-part-main-causes.aspx.

of healthcare resources among non-physicians. Burnout is a real, damaging, or potentially deadly problem throughout the world in varying degrees.

KEY BURNOUT DRIVERS

1. Loss of autonomy/employment
2. EMR (Electronic Medical Record)
3. Perverse incentives

LOSS OF AUTONOMY

The rise in burnout has paralleled the rise in physician employment by large organizations. We have lost our autonomy and the ability to control our destiny, work environment, hours, pay, and avoidance of hot-button issues by becoming employed by large healthcare institutions. In 1983, 76 percent of physicians owned their own practices. In 2016, for the first time ever, the percentage dropped below 50 percent, to 47.1 percent.[17]

In other words, physicians had, by a majority, given up their ability to be in control of their business, career, and life. Large healthcare systems, multispecialty clinics, hospitals, or even health insurance companies are now the employers of physicians. New policies and procedures are implemented. The day-to-day variability and control of physician practice has been outsourced to an employer. Their goals may or may not be the same as the physicians'.

This loss of control leads to increasing frustration over

---

17   Carol K. Kane, *Policy Research Perspectives: Updated Data on Physician Practice Arrangements: Physician Ownership Drops Below 50 Percent* (Chicago: American Medical Association, 2016).

being told how many patients to see, how many RVUs (relative value units, or work units) to produce, and how much vacation to take. Ultimately, these determine your income doing a stressful, complex, and sometimes dangerous job at all hours of the day and night.

Becoming employed can also lead to a situation where the coding, or assessment of what you do and the value of your work, is outsourced to a billing department. If their assessment of your work and coding is less than yours, you will automatically have to do more work to generate the same revenue. And the sum of loss of control and frustration, left at a low boil for years, turns into burnout.

EMR

The adoption of electronic medical record (EMR) systems has increased rapidly over the last ten to fifteen years, from 23 percent in 2003 to 69.6 percent in 2018.[18] Coincidentally, this parallels the rise in physician employment and the rise in burnout as well. EMR adoption was driven primarily by the Health Information Technology for Economic and Clinical Health (HITECH) Act of 2009 and the EMR component of the 2010 Affordable Care Act (ACA). Doctors and medical practices were first incentivized by supplemental payments, maximally $44,000 to $63,750 per physician, from the government to ease the cost burden of adopting these systems. These can cost sometimes as much as $50,000 to $100,000 per physician user.

---

18 Ibid.

After this initial honeymoon period of adoption, the incentives turned to penalties for not complying with reporting data on a giant, ever-changing list of criteria. Many of the reporting criteria never seemed applicable or practical for my urology practice to report on, but we did the best we could. The penalties vary but could be hundreds of thousands or millions of dollars based on the size of the penalty and the size of the physician group. Additionally, the day-to-day costs of adopting EMRs, including additional staff to input data, extra computing power and technology, faster internet connections to process data, and lost productivity of physicians can be many multiples of the actual cost, into the hundreds of thousands of dollars per year.

Finally, EMR usability, even as recently as 2019, has not been fixed despite endless user feedback, causing numerous user workarounds to function. These EMR systems can actually slow the transmission of medical information.[19]

Research has confirmed my intuition that EMR utilization is a major driver of burnout.[20] A recent study looked at the amount of time a group of family practice physicians interacted or used their EMR. In an 11.4-hour day, physicians interacted or used their EMR 355 minutes or nearly six hours. Half of the time, these doctors were working in one day, without emergencies or other responsibilities, was being used interacting with the system that, to date,

---

19 S. Assis-Hassid , B. J. Grosz, E. Zimlichman, R. Rozenblum, and D. W. Bates, "Assessing EHR Use during Hospital Morning Rounds: A Multifaceted Study," *PLoS ONE* 14, no. 2 (2019).

20 *Canadian Medical Association Journal* 189, no. 45 (November 13, 2017): E1405–E1406.

has never been proven in a randomized study to improve patient care.[21]

In my practice, we made the conscious decision to not have any screens in the patient rooms, so we cannot possibly be distracted by them for the patient experience. Does this mean it takes us longer outside the room to complete the record? Yes. But I refuse to give less than myself and my full attention to my patients. In my own research, 100 percent of survey respondents classify EMRs as a significant driver of their burnout, compared to 0 percent for seeing patients in clinic and 15 percent for doing surgery or procedures.

I have practiced during my career about 50 percent pre- and 50 percent post-EMR. I never felt the time scarcity and click pressure before EMR that I do now. Strictly from a time standpoint, I used to spend about thirty to forty minutes per day documenting all of my patient encounters. I now spend at least triple that amount of time and that is with offloading 75 percent of the data entry duties to our medical assistants, using speech recognition software and, realistically, shortening my face-to-face patient contact time to devote more time to documentation with the EMR.

Why do we use point-and-click systems that bring data input to a crawl? The time efficiency of knowledge and decision transmission has not improved in fifty-plus years in spite of EMRs. The lack of interoperability of EMRs has created a siloed medical information environment

21   B. G. Arndt et al., "Tethered to the EHR: Primary Care Physician Workload Assessment Using EHR Event Log Data and Time-Motion Observations," *Annals of Family Medicine* 15, no. 5 (2017): 419–426. doi: 10.1370/afm.2121.

that we have not unraveled yet. Fax technology, which was the first "push" technology, was the last real advance in medical information transmission, and that was more than forty years ago.

Those "push" information systems, where the data I need to do my job is automatically sent to me, far exceed the ease of use of disparate "pull" systems. In those "pull" systems, I now have to direct my staff to go get or pull that information from five, ten, or even more different systems, costing time, money, and care efficiency. There are attempts to create regional healthcare-information-sharing organizations, but they are classically incomplete, reducing usability and creating uncertainty about what I am missing and do not know about a patient. It is possible all of the patient's information is not represented by input from multiple physicians, labs, imaging, pathology labs, or hospital entities that may or may not participate in the regional health information warehouse.

It makes economic sense that we should take our highest value asset and use that asset to perform tasks and work that only that asset can do. We are heading toward a physician shortage by 2025, and it is estimated that by 2032 there will be a 122,000 physician shortage.[22] Would there be a doctor shortage if we had a system that allowed us to see 50–100 percent more patients in an efficient, easy, stress-free manner and not waste 50 percent of our time interacting with an EMR? Absolutely not. The precious natural resources of physician mental capacity, time, and energy are being squandered.

---

22 Association of American Medical Colleges, "The Complexities of Physician Supply and Demand: Projections from 2017–2032," April 2019.

PERVERSE INCENTIVES

A compounding driver of burnout is misaligned or perverse incentives. These lead to financial disincentives for doing the right thing for patients. In medicine, we are sometimes rewarded for inefficient care and penalized for efficient care. A frequent example for me is kidney stones. We receive calls from the emergency room about patients with symptomatic stones too large for the patient to pass spontaneously. We call it "the daily stone," as it is a common, essentially daily occurrence. A quick, easy way to temporize the situation and get the patient feeling better is to put in a stent, or internal drainage tube to drain the kidney. This, however, commits the patient to another surgery for the stone removal.

The other option is a longer, more difficult procedure to actually remove the stone which, depending on the size and location, may be a one- to two-hour procedure, unplanned, at the end of an already long day. What is best for the patient is one procedure if possible. But what is best for the physician, financially, is two procedures. I always pick one procedure if technically possible, clinically safe, and efficacious. But I know of doctors who feel it is best to always place a stent and return for a second procedure. Really, there is never a time where a patient's stone can be treated in one setting? Really? I am penalized, economically, for doing the right thing once. The other doctor is economically rewarded, twice for two procedures.

I have even heard of physicians who perform three procedures to take care of patients' stones. Wow! That seems incredible! Every single patient every time needs three procedures? Those doctors must live in an area with the most surgically complex stone patients ever.

By doing one procedure, if possible, I think I am way ahead, karma-wise, as well as advancing patient safety and convenience while decreasing cost and risk. I am saving the patient a second procedure, another anesthetic, and his/her insurance company $5,000–$10,000 or more in total expenditures. The patients really do appreciate it. In any other field, efficiency is rewarded. I should get a bonus for going the extra mile and taking care of this problem in one fell swoop. But no. There is no efficient-care bonus. This is just one small example of the malaligned incentives in medicine. The way the system fails to reward its users for an aligned effort leads to my frustration and, not surprisingly, burnout.

BURNOUT: A RESULT, NOT AN EFFECT

Becoming or being burned out is an end result, not a cause. Just as a heart attack is the result of genetics, diet, environment, toxins, and other factors, burnout is the culmination of multiple factors, leading to an event and/or a result that is usually unfavorable. These could include anger, resentment, compassion fatigue, increased medical errors, decreased empathy, workplace behavior outbursts, decreased or no work satisfaction, risk taking, substance abuse, depression, and even suicide.

Pamela Wible, MD, is a national expert on physician suicide. She runs her own practice but also serves as a de facto suicide prevention hotline for physicians. She has kept her own suicide registry of more than 1,300 physician and medical student suicides that she knows of in the last ten years. Physicians have the highest rate of suicide as a profession. During the writing of this book, one of my favorite doctors whom I have ever known committed suicide. Almost no mention of this was made of it by his group or the hospital. I met a doctor at a conference recently and she told me one of her partners and one of her residents in training had committed suicide in the last eighteen months.

It is estimated that the equivalent of one entire medical school or four hundred physicians per year commits suicide.[23] Physicians have two to four times the national rate of suicide attempts and, because we like to excel at everything, have a much higher rate of successful attempts as well. Male physicians are 40 percent more likely than the general population to commit suicide.[24] Female physicians are at even higher risk, at nearly 2.3 times the general population.[25] [26]

I had moments of suicidal ideation before treating my burnout. I never had a plan, but I got to the point where I wondered if things would simply be better if I just wasn't around. That was probably my personal low point. As soon as I had that thought, an electric shock went through me that made me realize what I did have. Suicide seemed like a permanent, selfish solution to temporary, fixable prob-

23   D. A. Sargent, V. W. Jensen, T. A. Petty, and H. Raskin, "Preventing Physician Suicide: The Role of Family, Colleagues, and Organized Medicine," *Journal of the American Medical Association* 237, no. 2 (January 10, 1977): 143–145.

24   E. S. Schernhammer and G. A. Colditz, "Suicide Rates among Physicians: A Quantitative and Gender Assessment (Meta-Analysis)," *American Journal of Psychiatry* 161, no. 12 (2004): 2295–2302. doi: 10.1176/appi.ajp.161.12.2295.

25   Ibid.

26   E. Frank and A. D. Dingle, "Self-Reported Depression and Suicide Attempts among U.S. Women Physicians," *American Journal of Psychiatry* 156, no. 12 (December 1999): 1887–1894.

lems. Escaping the trap of my circular, self-destructive thinking was a first step on recovery from burnout.

The current state of medicine is a public health crisis. No job or career is worth suicide. We know the definition and scope of burnout for our vocation and where that leaves us: in deep trouble.

HOW DID WE GET HERE, INDIVIDUALLY AND AS A PROFESSION?

HOW DID I GET HERE?

Before and during medical school, you will do just about whatever it takes to get in and succeed, without regard for your personal well-being, health, life, or other goals. That early lesson in denying care for yourself presages what comes next and is really the first brick in the burnout wall. Residency then becomes a paying (residents are paid to work and learn) medical school on steroids. You are essentially a highly educated medieval serf, rented out to the institution to which you are employed.

During the pre-empathy epoch in which I trained, the attitude toward work was, get it done no matter what it takes. Work one hundred hours per week? No problem. Work 120 hours per week? Still no problem. Work six months without a day off? Piece of cake. Take every-other-night in-house call (sleeping in the hospital) for two years? Are you kidding? You miss half of the pathology on your night off. No one wants to be labeled "lazy" or, even worse, "weak." My worst week during my internship: I worked 140 hours. There are only 168 hours in a week.

If that work schedule does not beat into your head that you and your life are always assumed to come in second place to medicine, I do not know what will. This work ethic, while impressive and nearly psychotic, has been recently shown to cause actual genetic damage by increasing the rate of telomere shortening by six- to twenty-five-fold in medical residents during training.[27] Shorter telomeres are related to shorter life spans.[28]

Common sense and some horrible outcomes from sleep-deprived residents caring for patients stimulated reforms for resident workload, weekly work-hour restrictions, and actually treating residents like human beings. Those changes occurred after my residency. I am told the work-hour restrictions may not work as intended. But the pressure to conform to fairly inhuman work expectations still exists.

Residency is where the conditioning continues, teaching you to take whatever the system deals out, which can be a lot of bullshit. In response to the never-ending demands, I developed several concepts related to bullshit, which we will explore more in chapter 11. First, there was the Bull-shit Bucket. That was the absolute maximum of what BS I would tolerate and take before I would fight back, take a stand, or change my environment. There were definite times in my residency where I had taken all I could take and I was not going to take any more.

But, unfortunately, I had a very large BS bucket, so it took

27 https://doi.org/10.1016/j.biopsych.2019.04.030

28 *Proceedings of the National Academy of Sciences of the United States* 116, no. 30 (July 23, 2019): 15122–15127.

a lot to fill it. It was and is a balancing act between being a "team player" and a pushover as far as what BS you are willing to accept. Perhaps this was my first reaction to burnout or my particular line in the sand across which I could not be pushed when my bucket got full. The problem now is that the filling of the bucket never stops, the patient flow continues and the endless ratcheting up of regulations, mouse clicks, and medically necessary (but clinically useless) documentation continues without a way to counteract it. You define what BS you let into your bucket and the quantity.

Second, I originated the concept of the Benefit-Bullshit Ratio. This is a purely subjective evaluation by me of the ratio of good things over bad things. For example, you might count good events or compliments from patients on the top of the ratio over irritating and frustrating occurrences. You could count "good days" over "bad days." It's up to you. Once the ratio starts to dip below three, it may be time to make some changes. It is sometimes difficult to see where the benefits are today, so the ratio sometimes dips below one. This is clearly not satisfactory long term.

Residency is also where the work itself may cause burnout, as the sheer number of hours spent at the hospital, caring for patients, dealing with staff, nurses, and medical students wear you down. But the true, exquisite nature of burnout comes only after you finish residency. Here, the professional demands exceed your expectation of an improving life as well as your time, energy, and emotional ability to overcome those demands.

Medical training feels like a series of ladders, climbing to the top of one, then starting over at the bottom rung of the next one—applicant to medical school, admitted to medical school, first-year medical student, rising to an M4 (fourth-year medical student), only to be knocked back to the bottom as an intern, then to R2 (second-year resident), then to chief resident.

Academic medicine would have been a career possibility for me but would have meant another ladder, starting with assistant professor, then associate professor, then professor, chair, dean...and ultimately, I think, God.

I thought private practice would be an escape from this endless climb. And to a certain extent, that is true, as there are really only two types of doctors in private practice—employees and partners or owners. As a physician employee, you do the work, get paid a salary and maybe bonuses, and go home. As an employee, there are no worries about running a small business, personnel issues, payroll, overhead, and the million other day-to-day decisions.

As an owner, partner, or associate, you own and run the business or hire someone to do that for you. Private practice is a small business, and like any other business, it requires, at a minimum, some strategic guidance and oversight by the owners. This comes along with all the headaches and benefits of small business ownership: personnel, insurance, contracting, management, taxes, compliance, regulatory knowledge, strategy, pro formas of new opportunities, cash flow, paying yourself last, and so many more joys and opportunities. By the way, none of those skills are taught in medical school.

I learned that how good I am as a doctor has a very small impact on my success. My success as a practitioner has more to do with availability, affability, and ability. It seemed ability was the least important at times. Patient referral patterns, community visibility, and patient accessibility, sometimes regardless of the quality and level of care, can trump skill and knowledge. It's not what you know but who you know and how easy it is for patients to see you.

After learning a financially painful vocabulary lesson around tax time on the definition of "net income," I became much more involved in the management of my practice. It took only an hour or two per day of my time for the last twenty years—for which I asked my partners no further compensation—but I directed activities and made decisions that made or saved millions of dollars to our collective bottom line. Should I have asked for compensation for the value I brought to my practice? Yes. Shame on me for not? Yes. But chapter closed. I am a big believer that I cannot change the past, but I can move forward from where I am now. Running harder every day for less enjoyment and revenue with more frustration led me to the final event in my crispification burnout process—my cracked keyboard and its untimely demise. I was burned out!

HOW DID WE GET HERE AS A PROFESSION?

There are a few reasons why medicine has now found itself at a crossroads. Increasing expectations, cognitive mismatches, and workplace stress all contribute to where we are. But let's take the pulse of medicine, statistically, and see how it is doing. Nearly half of its practitioners are burning out and one out of seven are suicidal.[29] Seventy percent of doctors would not recommend healthcare as a profession.[30] Large studies over the last ten years have shown burnout rates to be 45 percent in 2011, 54 percent in 2014, and falling to 44 percent in 2017.[31] [32] A 2018 survey showed that 67 percent of urologists are either burned out or becoming burned out. Twenty-five percent are making active plans to leave urology in the next two years.[33] And, while I know all physicians are overachievers, as a urologist, I hate to be the number one specialty for rates of burnout for 2019.[34] (See graphic below.) If the statistics above were vital signs, you might say that medicine is on life support.

29 *Medscape National Physician Burnout, Depression and Suicide Report 2019.*

30 The Doctors Company, *The Future of Healthcare: A National Survey of Physicians—2018.*

31 Tait D. Shanafelt et al., "Changes in Burnout and Satisfaction with Work-Life Balance in Physicians and the General US Working Population between 2011 and 2014," *Mayo Clinic Proceedings* 90, no. 12 (2015): 1600–1613.

32 Tait D. Shanafelt et al., "Changes in Burnout and Satisfaction with Work-Life Integration in Physicians and the General US Working Population between 2011 and 2017," *Mayo Clinic Proceedings* 94, no. 9 (2019): 1681–1694. doi: 10.1016/j.mayocp.2018.10.023.

33 *Urology Times*, December 2018, pp. 1, 22.

34 *Medscape National Physician Burnout, Depression & Suicide Report 2019*, slide 3.

Which Physicians Are Most Burned Out?

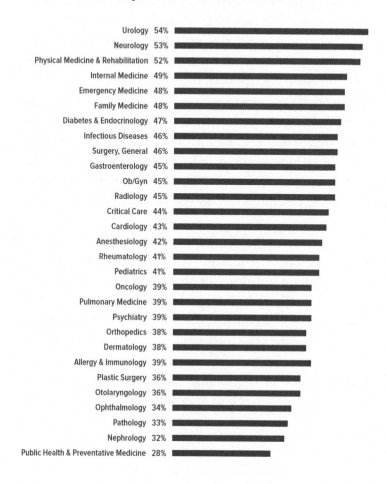

Specialty	Percentage
Urology	54%
Neurology	53%
Physical Medicine & Rehabilitation	52%
Internal Medicine	49%
Emergency Medicine	48%
Family Medicine	48%
Diabetes & Endocrinology	47%
Infectious Diseases	46%
Surgery, General	46%
Gastroenterology	45%
Ob/Gyn	45%
Radiology	45%
Critical Care	44%
Cardiology	43%
Anesthesiology	42%
Rheumatology	41%
Pediatrics	41%
Oncology	39%
Pulmonary Medicine	39%
Psychiatry	39%
Orthopedics	38%
Dermatology	38%
Allergy & Immunology	39%
Plastic Surgery	36%
Otolaryngology	36%
Ophthalmology	34%
Pathology	33%
Nephrology	32%
Public Health & Preventative Medicine	28%

Burnout is also associated with increased medical errors and malpractice risk.[35] In fact, the risk of perceived medical errors by physicians can be quantitated to a 4 percent increased risk for every night of call duty.[36] [37] In a recent review, more than two-thirds of studies looking at burnout saw increasing medical errors with burned-out physicians.[38] And the rate of medical errors may be triple that of non-burned-out physicians.[39] An ICU study showed an increased mortality rate for patients cared for by burned-out physicians. Not only is burnout dangerous for physicians, but it can also be deadly for patients.

In strictly economic terms, burnout is an expensive proposition. A burned-out physician costs between $500,000 and $1 million to replace, or up to two to three times their salary.[40] The costs have been studied at Stanford University, where they estimate potential annual expenditures for replacement of burned-out physicians at greater than $5 million.[41] These losses do not account for any detrimental health or well-being effects for the physician or institutional loss, such as leadership experience or capa-

35   C. M. Balch et al., "Personal Consequences of Malpractice Lawsuits on American Surgeons," *Journal of the American College of Surgeons* 213 (2011): 657–667.

36   L. H. Hall, J. Johnson, I. Watt, A. Tsipa, and D. B. O'Connor, "Healthcare Staff Wellbeing, Burnout, and Patient Safety: A Systematic Review," *PLoS One* 11, no. 7 (2016): e0159015.

37   Tait D. Shanafelt et al., "Burnout and Medical Errors among American Surgeons," *Annals of Surgery* 251, no. 6 (June 2010): 995–1000.

38   Hall et al., "Healthcare Staff Wellbeing, Burnout, and Patient Safety."

39   T. Shanafelt et al., "Physician Burnout, Well-Being, and Work Unit Safety Grades in Relationship to Reported Medical Errors," *Mayo Clinic Proceedings* 93, no. 11 (November 2018): 1571–1580.

40   *JAMA Internal Medicine* 177, no. 12 (2017): 1826–1832.

41   S. Berg, "At Stanford, Physician Burnout Costs At Least $7.75 Million a Year," *JAMA News*, November 17, 2017.

bilities that also leave with the burned-out physician. A burned-out physician is much more likely to transition to part-time work in the next several years after burnout peaks.[42] To be sure, burnout is bad for business.

INCREASING EXPECTATIONS

The rapid evolution of medicine has led to a nearly impossible trifecta of new patient care demands, new information technology, and poor workflow for physicians. These occurred without new tools to achieve the tasks at hand. A large problem that arises now is cognitive and expectation dissonance, or what I like to call mismatches. There are mismatches in empathy, expectations, and the current set of tools available to physicians and the type of work being done.

MISMATCH: EMPATHY

Over the past forty to fifty years, there was an increasing emphasis in medicine on cutting-edge technologies, new medicines, and surgical procedures. As technology increased, bedside manner may have suffered in the interim. Patients felt a loss of connection with their doctor, or "provider." Seeing this decline in empathy and compassion[43] for the last ten to fifteen years, medical schools have refocused on training the "whole doctor" with new and additional classes in sensitivity training, interpersonal skills, and empathy.[44] In actuality, empathy is a trait that

---

42 *Mayo Clinic Proceedings* 91, no. 4: 422–431.

43 *Academic Medicine* 84, no. 9 (September 2009): 1182–1191.

44 https://www.huffingtonpost.com/antonio-m-gotto-jr-md-dphil/teaching-empathy-in-medic_b_3867262.html

can be enhanced or taught, as "cognition and understanding (the prominent ingredients of empathy) can be substantially enhanced by education."[45] That learning may or may not be occurring, but the simple fact that empathy now has to be taught, and cannot be demonstrated, modeled, or mentored as previously, is concerning. Doctors are always caring about others first, so we output our thoughts, feelings, needs, and desires second, after we fulfill the need or obligation at hand. Most humans operate 100 percent of their time on earth in their own best interests. As a job requirement, being a physician begins with the consideration of another's interests. This can be counterintuitive and exhausting over time if a physician does not spend enough time "considering" him- or herself.

MISMATCH: EXPECTATION VS. TOOLS AVAILABLE

The expectations by patients, institutions, and payers for physician performance are sky high on all levels and metrics. We are expected to be "Super Doctor." Between payer "report cards" on my efficiency (or really, my cost to them), bad Google reviews for patients waiting five minutes to see me while I am saving someone else's life, medical board scrutiny, the federal Physician Payments Sunshine Act (for which we are compelled to be accountable for how many pretzels we may have eaten at a pharmaceutical-sponsored event), expectations and complete transparency of my practice and life have never been higher. It is fairly exhausting just trying to keep up with what you are trying to comply with while helping patients.

---

45 *Academic Medicine* 84, no. 9 (September 2009): 1183.

The tools or processes I am forced to use daily are not designed to maximize care for the patient, contrary to my wishful expectations. When I am sitting in front of a patient, assessing the facts, symptoms, exam, lab results, and all available data, I believe that I am best equipped to make an appropriate decision for care, evaluation, or therapy. That appears to be a foolish assumption according to the patient's insurance company and their protocols.

For example, when I think a patient in pain needs a CT scan to look for a problem, I will order it. Ten to twenty percent of the time, a person from the insurance company with apparently no greater than a high school education has a list of protocols and diagnoses for which they can approve a CT scan. They mispronounce this list of diagnoses as they tell me the study I want to order may or may not be covered by that particular insurance unless they receive the dreaded "more documentation" of the need for the study.

We submit the requested extra information. Hours to days go by. My patient is still in pain. Then, if the CT is still not approved by the payer, I get to escalate the process to do a peer review with a doctor, almost never a urologist, to discuss the medical necessity of this particular CT scan. More days go by. My patient is still in pain and now may be going to the most expensive place in the universe to obtain care—the emergency room.

This would seem to defeat the cost savings of the precertification process. I do have an ultimate fallback position for this process of approval. I tell the peer-review doctor that if they come to my office, examine the patient, and write a note in my chart that, in their medical opinion, this patient does not need a CT, then I will be fine with their decision. Of course, as a non-urological specialist employed by the health insurance company and sitting in an office one thousand miles away, the doctor will not do that, and my request for a CT is approved. I have 100 percent success with this technique for study approval. However, what a silly, time-wasting game to go through to still approve a study I ordered now days or weeks ago!

The vast majority of physicians went to medical school to care for patients, not become scribes, data entry clerks, debate jousting experts with peer reviewers, or editors of twelve-page notes that contain no useful information. A useful exercise would be for the healthcare industry to improve all medical processes and focus on what is best for caring for the patient, easy to do and efficient for those providing the care.

MISMATCH: BUSYWORK

The final mismatch is between what makes intuitive medical sense and what is useless busywork. I am completely prepared, mentally at peace, and trained to get out of bed at one in the morning to operate on someone to save their life (a very good thing!). I am not prepared, at peace, or trained to click forty-seven boxes in an EMR to fulfill "meaningful use" requirements devised by someone twelve states away who has never cared for a patient, with a process that does not improve patient care. And the amount of work needed by me to complete my EMR tasks is two to five times more in the United States than anywhere else in the entire world.[46]

---

46 *Annals of Internal Medicine* 169, no. 1 (2018): 50–51.

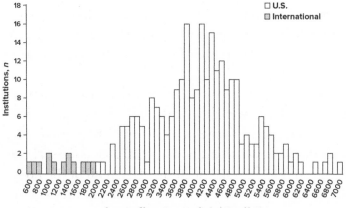

Average Characters per Ambulatory Note, n

It is this unnecessary extra work that increases stress in the workplace. Dr. Jeffrey Pfeffer is a professor of organizational behavior at the Graduate School of Business at Stanford University. He has extensively studied workplace stress, its negative health and productivity impacts, and organizational changes in the workplace to mitigate its effects. In a recent *Wall Street Journal* article,[47] Pfeffer suggests three strategies for employers to decrease employee workplace stress: regular, limited work hours, greater autonomy, and more economic security.

Pfeffer found that implementing these strategies reduced employee stress and healthcare costs, while increasing productivity, health, and well-being. That is very encouraging and forward thinking.

The only problem? In medical workplaces, very few of these strategies are employed, and actually we appear to be going backward on all three fronts. We now have longer, more irregular hours, decreased autonomy, and perhaps the least

---

47   *The Wall Street Journal*, March 2–3, 2019, p. C3.

amount of economic security ever, as more physicians serve at the whims of an employer instead of being self-employed. Why does the medical system care least for the care providers?

There are limits to the nonclinical tasks, the deteriorating workplace environment, and the lack of value for aligned effort that can be asked of a doctor without increasing resentment, frustration, and burnout. That is the real crux of burnout for physicians today. Given all of the above, the myth of the Super Doctor is fraying at the edges or has torn completely. We simply cannot do it all anymore. Burnout has proven to be an increasing phenomenon and can result in expensive, error-prone, harmful, potentially deadly, time- and resource-wasting care.

How do we refute Mr. Dostoevsky's assertion that you will burn out? How do we avoid burnout? By first determining if we are, in fact, burned out.

CHAPTER 2 TAKEAWAYS

- Burnout is defined as emotional exhaustion, depersonalization, and diminished personal accomplishment.
- Burnout is a worldwide, universal worker phenomenon.
- Key drivers of burnout are loss of autonomy, EMR, and perverse incentives.
- Physician suicide is a national health crisis.
- Consider your BS Bucket and your Benefit-BS ratio.
- Physicians are burned out at high, dangerous, costly levels.
- Burnout increases the risk of medical errors and malpractice.
- Systemic forces increase burnout.

CHAPTER 3

Are You Burned Out?

"We all crash and burn. Some of us just burn a little brighter."
— CURTIS TYRONE JONES

The title of this chapter could be "I Was a Bad Dad." Over the last twenty years, I definitely made choices that prioritized work, business, and my medical practice over time with my family. I was so frustrated and angry with the state of medicine and the state of my practice that I felt if I worked harder, something would be better that would improve my life. This may have just been tilting at windmills. And not surprisingly, more time at work and away from my family did not actually improve either. Have you ever felt that you had made efforts that yielded few or no results? How did that make you feel? I became even more frustrated, hopeless, and confused when this happened. This was nearly a daily occurrence for me.

In retrospect, which is always 20/20, the decisions I made to never coach any of my kids' sports teams, spend more time with them, or always be home every night for dinner and/or bedtime were not the right choices. Have you made choices that prioritized work over family and life? Is that a recurrent theme? One of my colleagues related to me that she was a parent and a doctor but always felt she was "sucking at both" of those jobs. There are competing, impossible demands.

I am trying to rectify this now by definitely being more present when I'm with my wife and my kids. I am trying to be more interactive with them on a regular basis. I have a fabulous wife and some of the nicest, sweetest, coolest kids that I have ever met. I am endeavoring to improve those relationships. Every day is another chance for you to make those changes in your life.

BURNOUT SURVEYS AND QUESTIONS

At this point, you may have taken all the burnout questionnaires (Maslach Burnout Inventory,[48] Mayo Clinic Well-Being Index,[49] Physician Well-Being Index,[50] Mental Health Association Stress Screener[51]), passed the medical board inquisition about your mental health, and are certain you are not burned out! Great! You may not be getting a little crispy around the edges, but ask yourself some of these questions:

Have you ever been frustrated by the late patient when you are desperately trying to get out of the office to make it to a concert, play, dinner, sporting event, or life?

---

48   https://www.mindgarden.com/117-maslach-burnout-inventory

49   https://www.mayo.edu/research/centers-programs/program-physician-well-being/
     mayos-approach-physician-well-being/mayo-clinic-well-being-index

50   https://www.mededwebs.com/well-being-index/physician-well-being-index

51   https://www.mhanational.org/get-involved/stress-screened

Have you ever wished that an end-stage patient who is only suffering would be let go by their family?

Have you wondered why you do what you do, and if it is worth what you are giving?

If you have positive responses to any of those questions, then you may be in the first stages of burnout, especially if these thoughts or feelings occur more than just at the end of a bad day, or at 10:00 p.m., when you are still finishing your electronic charts.

Other areas in which you may be exhibiting symptoms of burnout may include:

- **Social/mental/physical health:** Are you stressed, overworked, underexercised, malnourished, in relationship 911, angry, frustrated, or overmedicated for sleep, anxiety, or irritability?
- **Work performance:** Do you have poor productivity, errors, lack of timeliness of records, poor patient and/ or colleague communication?
- **Relationships:** Are you seeing declines in your satisfaction personally and professionally with colleagues and staff? Are you seeing increasing patient complaints? Has your Google rating fallen?
- **Professional associations:** Have you lost privileges or been suspended from board certification, hospitals, or insurance panels?
- **Medical health:** Have you under- or not treated your own hypertension, diabetes, weight gain, insomnia, depression because "you don't have time"?
- **Financial:** Have you been rushed in decision making,

had poor money management, poor focus on finances, impulsivity, scarcity of money, late fees on bills, poor or nonexistent tax or estate planning?

- **Clinical:** Do you have responsibilities that take all your time and provide no benefit? Examples could be call coverage, EMR, documentation, committees, or administrative tasks.

A positive response to any one or a constellation of these questions may be the first signs of burnout. Be aware they exist, and use them as cautions going forward. Understand that you are not only your job or work situation. That is a small part of your life. When we focus only on work and when work goes badly, our ability to maintain perspective, balance, and functionality declines.

THE DOCTOR MINDSET AS THE BURNOUT MINDSET?

People would like to think of themselves as an identity or construct and that we are "done": "I finished medical school and residency. I am now a doctor." That is a convenient way to live life. It saves mental energy and is a productive paradigm with which to interpret, plan, and respond to life. And, yes, that is part of your identity. When things are going well with that mindset, hooray! It works well and there is not much to worry about.

But the mistake made is when that becomes a fixed perception or mindset. When changes, especially negative ones such as burnout, occur, that fixed mindset does not allow for new ways of thinking, introspection, problem solving, option generation, empowerment, or hope. You are not a cake. You will never be fully baked or "done." You, as a person, are under constant evolution. You just may not realize that yet. Allow yourself to change, adapt, learn, and improve. All of those skills will help with burnout recovery.

Burnout does in fact incorporate emotional exhaustion, depersonalization, and decreased personal accomplishment. I would like to add two other components to my pretreatment burnout constellation of symptoms: powerlessness and hopelessness. Not only does burnout drain your energy to deal with day-to-day demands, but it seems to also instill a sense of permanence about your current situation or emotional state and a sense of futility about possible changes. Prior to diagnosing and treating myself, I was convinced that my work life was horrible, and more significantly, there was nothing I could do about it. That boxed-in mentality only exacerbated my other burnout symptoms. It created a sense of imprisonment.

Just as a fish cannot be asked what water is because of lack of perspective, a person in burnout may not realize they are burning out. That is why asking the question, "Am I burned out?" may be your first step to diagnosis and recovery. Remember that dictum from medical school: The only diagnosis you can't make is the one you don't consider. Consider the possibility that you have burnout.

Fortunately, I have been reassured by my kids that I was not a bad dad. But it is time to recognize that we all can burn out, with the question of how brightly we burn. Let's address how to treat burnout by knowing where we are going.

CHAPTER 3 TAKEAWAYS

- Question yourself about areas of frustration in your life. These may indicate burnout.
- Your self-perception is not fixed.
- You are not powerless or hopeless.
- Open your mind to other options.
- Consider the possibility of burnout as a diagnosis for you.

CHAPTER 4

Where Are You Going?

"If you don't know where you want to go, any road will get you there."

—LEWIS CARROLL, *ALICE IN WONDERLAND*

Starting a journey without any particular destination in mind is a recipe for lots of wasted time, effort, and resources and will end in even more frustration than you are feeling now. It is critical we know where we are going. There are many possible paths you can take to diagnose and treat your burnout. Let's explore your possible routes to less burnout and a better life. But before we propose potentially new or different treatment strategies for burnout, we should assess current therapeutic options and strategies. However, those solutions may not be reaching or helping the intended audience with the desired impact.

The standard therapy typically involves improving physician-related factors as well as organizational, or healthcare system, factors. Improving organizational factors has actually been shown to be more important for improving burnout for physicians.[52] But the best solutions for burn-

---

52   N. Lown et al., "Resilience: What Is It, Why Do We Need It, and Can It Help Us?" *British Journal of General Practice* 65, no. 639 (2015): e708–e710. doi: 10.3399/bjgp15X687133.

out combine both personal and institutional improvement strategies. Working on all fronts, as detailed throughout the rest of this book, will bring you the best results.

CURRENT INSTITUTIONAL SOLUTIONS

The Mayo Clinic has been a national leader in evaluation and treatment strategies for burnout. They have a large employed-physician group with which to evaluate, survey, test, and implement interventions.

The nine strategies the Mayo Clinic suggests organizations should begin to resolve burnout are:

1. Acknowledging and assessing the problem.
2. Recognizing the behaviors of leaders that can increase or decrease burnout.
3. Using a systems approach to develop targeted interventions to improve efficiency and reduce clerical work.
4. Cultivating community at work.
5. Using rewards and incentives strategically.
6. Assessing whether the organization's actions are aligned with the stated values and mission.
7. Implementing organizational practices and policies that promote flexibility and work-life balance.
8. Providing resources to help individuals promote self-care.
9. Supporting organizational science or study factors in your own institution that contribute to the problem and invest in solutions.[53]

---

53 Mayo Clinic, "Mayo Clinic: Reversing Physician Burnout, Using Nine Strategies to Promote Well-Being, 2016," https://newsnetwork.mayoclinic.org/discussion/ mayo-clinic-reversing-physician-burnout-using-nine-strategies-to-promote-well-being/.

I agree with all of those steps. But for the 40–50 percent of physicians in this country without a staff, budget, or chief wellness officer to aid them, this book aims to fill that gap.

The American Medical Association has also been a leader in advocating for improving conditions for physicians. In its Steps Forward Module, the AMA has a well-documented action plan to address physician burnout and create more satisfied and productive physicians. These steps include:

CREATING A CULTURE OF WELLNESS:

1. Engage senior leadership.
2. Track the business case for well-being.
3. Resource a wellness infrastructure.
4. Measure wellness and the predictors of burnout longitudinally.
5. Strengthen local leadership.
6. Develop and evaluate interventions.

CREATING AN EFFICIENCY OF PRACTICE:

1. Develop and evaluate interventions.
2. Reduce clerical burden and tame the EHR and *creating personal resilience.*
3. Support the physical and psychosocial health of the workforce.[54]

These again are all admirable goals and do give an outline for moving forward. The details seem to be left to the

---

54 American Medical Association, "STEPS in Practice," 2018, https://www.stepsforward.org/modules/joy-in-medicine.

individual. Action steps are hard to find for that burned-out individual and harder to implement. Sometimes, even the best current solutions like those detailed above lack specifics and a path to follow.

RESILIENCE

A component of many early burnout treatment programs was resiliency training. The focus is typically on how to better deal with your situation, meditate, and accept what you cannot change. There is definitely a place for improvement by using resiliency training and coping mechanisms. I am an example of those (see chapter 19). However, I didn't seem to need resiliency training ten or twenty years ago.

Can we get real about resilience for a second? It seems to be all the rage to talk about burnout and the ways that physicians can withstand burnout better with more resilience. As a physician, it would seem that if there is a problem, let's solve the problem, instead of liking it better or doing more deep breathing. If we followed the resilience paradigm in medicine, we would smile a lot more while cancer was killing our patients.

All physicians are resilient. Our jobs require us to evaluate dangerous, life-threatening situations, make snap decisions, and perform care swiftly and accurately. Then take a breath, refocus, and move on thirty seconds later to the next potential disaster. If that is not resilient, I don't know what is.

I was recently at a conference of physicians, where most of

the presenters were non-physicians. One of the physicians related a story of how he had finished an eighteen-hour shift before getting on the plane to come to the conference. Every non-physician in the room was completely astounded by this feat of diligence and dedication. Pretty much every physician there shrugged after hearing the story. "Only eighteen hours? At least you probably got to eat and maybe sleep before or after your work." Resilient? Hell, yeah! But your goddamn EMR and work environment are killing me.

Resiliency training without foundational institutional and personal changes sounds like deciding if a smaller bite or some barbecue sauce will make that stool sandwich you are eating go down a little better. By that, I mean, helping the burned-out cope with an increasingly impossible workload, time demands, and worsening workplace and malpractice environment does not fix those problems. It attempts to make us feel better about how bad things are.

Rather than choking down a stool sub sammie, I want to change the MENU! Instead of meekly and powerlessly accepting our lot in our medical life, let's open our minds to different paradigms, work and life structures, productivity metrics, and acceleration of development of tools that are helpful to physicians, not harmful.

BURNOUT TREATMENT OPTIONS

So where do we go? As I said at the beginning of this section, if you don't know where you want to go, any road will get you there. We now know what the definition of the problem is. What are our options for evaluation and treatment?

Here they are:

1. Ignore it. Suck it up. Rub some dirt on it. Bottle it up until it reaches a fine boil in the pressure cooker of your mind and body, and see how that goes. Not well, usually, and we are currently seeing the results of this method.
2. Try some very minor peripheral actions and techniques. Take a vacation. Meditate. Complain to your healthcare organization about changes with little response or no results. And try the ever-popular resiliency training.
3. Take a sabbatical. I know of at least three colleagues who are leaving medical practice for one to six months, traveling, living in other countries, and generally checking out of their current situation. They are being begged to come back as soon as possible by their healthcare organizations.
4. Drugs, alcohol, substance abuse. Avoidance of a problem is a technique but generally harmful for all involved and does not solve or change the problem.
5. Suicide is a permanent, painful, unnecessary solution to a temporary, fixable problem.
6. Seek care from a licensed, qualified psychologist!
7. Try the standard evaluation and treatment algorithms, which are possible first steps, if you can figure out how to initiate and implement them and have the resources.
8. Completely reevaluate everything about your life, work, decision-making process, personal and professional agreements that you have made, and your response to them. Evaluate what you have constructed as your life, and reconstruct a new, better, more meaningful one. This is what we advocate in this book and will guide you through that process and down the road to your goals to the new "you." We won't leave you, like Alice, taking any road with no particular destination.

CHAPTER 4 TAKEAWAYS

- Know where you are going.
- Standard therapies for burnout work best inside large, well-resourced systems.
- Hell, yes, you are resilient, but that is not the only tool in your toolbox!
- There are options for you going forward.
- Get ready to reevaluate your current life construct to build a new one.

PART II

Transitions

To get from where you are to where you want to go will require change. Taking chances and making changes require new ways of thinking and acting. That will lead to transitions in your life toward your new "you."

For burnout, this gets a little tricky, as we need to back up just a bit and talk about what you have done before you arrived at this point. In part, what has led you here are your agreements and your reasons for what you do. Fortunately, these are components of your life that are completely under your control. Let's get ready to change your thinking and change your life!

CHAPTER 5

Your Agreements

"No one can make you feel inferior without your consent."

—ELEANOR ROOSEVELT

Eleanor Roosevelt would have told you that no one can force an agreement on you without your consent as well. Your consent to agreements is a critical aspect of the construction of your life, the defining parameters of what you do and where you live. Everything in your life is, to a very large extent, a result of your own actions, reactions, and decisions in response to your agreements. You must accept, internalize, and take responsibility for this. Let's explore the process.

An agreement can be defined as:

1. A negotiated and typically legally binding arrangement between parties as to a course of action.
2. Harmony or accordance in opinion or feeling; a position or result of agreeing.
3. The absence of incompatibility between two things; consistency.[55]

---

55 https://en.oxforddictionaries.com/definition/us/agreement

As you can see, some agreements are written and explicit, some are felt or implied, and sometimes "agreement" simply means an absence of conflict. Whatever the meaning, agreements control our efforts and actions and our responses to events in our lives.

Understand that there is only one way you arrive at your current situation and that is with your assent, or lack of dissent. You have either said yes or did not say no to certain agreements.

You must accept responsibility for your current situation, which is really an accumulation of all the decisions, actions, and consent you have given or acceded to someone else. Your current outcomes and life are 100 percent of your own making. This is certain. No one forced your life on you.

Let me make this crystal clear: I am not blaming anyone. I just want everyone to accept their own role in the life/mess of their creation. If you are anything like me, you don't need another opportunity to feel bad about yourself. I am merely trying to point out that accepting personal responsibility and awareness are the first steps in making changes.

Thank God that you are responsible for your life and the decisions that led you here. That is wonderful because if you do not like where you are, all you need to do is to change your decisions and your agreements. This is why you are reading this book in the first place.

Life is a series of choices. I know there is a lot of popular psychology that may say that we are victims of circumstance, not choice. And we can blame everything on the baby boomers, or Generations X, Y, and Z, the millennials, or global warming for that matter. This outsources the control of our own lives to a locus outside of ourselves. I disagree. There are numerous examples of the worst possible situations in life that people have faced and they have overcome those circumstances to become happy, fulfilled, and successful. One of my friends was born without the ability to walk, is an Olympic gold medal winner, has been in a Nike commercial, and is one of the most incredible people I have ever met. You control your choices and that to which you agree.

What you agree to is what you accept, and that will form the basis of your life. All I am saying is that you should be very careful about that to which you agree. The decision process can take on a life of its own. This can be characterized by decision momentum. This is a term I use to describe the unrelenting train that we all seem to sometimes not be able to get off when making one or a series of decisions or agreements. Decision momentum can fuel consecutive good or bad agreements. "Well, I have already eaten one Oreo, so fifty-three more will be OK." "I have already spent ten years getting my medical degree and residency training, and even though I hate what I now do with a passion, I can't give up on my/my mom's/my dad's dream of being a doctor." There is a certain degree of decision momentum and/or herd mentality in medicine that lulls medical students, residents, and physicians into thinking that "if everybody else is doing it, it must be right/a good idea/the way it is." This can then turn one bad agreement into a series of errors. Controlling your agreements, one at a time, can prevent poor decision momentum.

There are different types of agreements. Some agreements

that you make with yourself are overt, loud, and obvious, such as applying for medical school, asking someone to marry you, or which burrito you order.

Others are more insidious and tacit, such as acquiescing to a pay gap between yourself and a less qualified, less productive, or gender-different partner. Or allowing a hospital to not give you the required resources to be a happy, productive physician because you don't want to rock the boat or cause extra expense, even though it will mean taking charts home every night for the rest of your career to "catch up."

Our lives are governed by our agreements. Yes, I agree to work hard, take the right classes, take the MCAT, apply and get into medical school. You agree to educate me and teach me what it takes to become a doctor. I agree to marry this beautiful person, which is a very nice agreement! I agree to pay my bills, work for X dollars in exchange for Y efforts.

YOUR AGREEMENTS

Do you know what your agreements are? Are you happy and contented with the agreements you have overtly or tacitly made?

Your agreements become giant sources of joy or pain in your life.

Let's list a few of your agreements below, then check either joy or pain. For example, "I agree to work fifty hours a week and take call." For me, that is both joy and pain, so I check both. "I agree to coach my daughter's soccer team!" JOY! And maybe a smidgen of pain...

Think about a few of your noncontractual agreements, such as "I will be home for dinner at least five nights a week," or "My spouse and I have date night once per week," or "I agree to go to therapy once per week to work on my issues." I would venture to guess that more than 90 percent of our agreements are not written down.

Get your favorite scribing instrument or device, and using the list below, write yours down—all of them, both overt and the tacit. This will give you a much better idea of the volume and scope of all of your agreements. And once they are written down, you get to decide if you still agree with them anymore.

AGREEMENTS	JOY	PAIN

_____ _____ _____

_____ _____ _____

_____ _____ _____

_____ _____ _____

_____ _____ _____

Ideally, you have far more or only "Joy" check marks. You may want to divide your agreements into sections such as Work, Mental, Physical/Heath, Financial, Spiritual, and Social categories to help organize them in your mind and on paper.

If you have many more "Pain" check marks, reassess what you are agreeing to, either tacitly or overtly. Decide the value and validity of those particular agreements. Some may be old and outdated. Some may be painful and unnecessary. Take this time to reassess what you are agreeing to, and take back control of your life. This is an important step. Eleanor Roosevelt would be proud of you and your control of your consent. Now that we know to what you have agreed, let's determine why you make those agreements.

CHAPTER 5 TAKEAWAYS

- Your agreements define your life with your consent or lack of dissent.
- You are responsible for your current set of agreements.
- Agreements bring joy or pain into your life.

- Write down your agreements and assess the joy or pain they bring you.
- Decide if you still value your previous agreements.

CHAPTER 6

Your Why

Bringing a New "You" into Being

"Where there is no vision, the people perish."

—PROVERBS 29:18

Nothing like a biblical reference to instill some foreboding, eh? Let's get you a vision and a way to your future and how to make those changes. First, we have to know your motivation for what you do, personally and professionally, or what your "why" is. As your "why" is a mental construct, either known or unknown to you, let's spend some time examining your thinking process, and ask some basic questions.

ORIENT YOURSELF

Where are you? What is your current, concrete situation? Employed, married, current locale?

Where are you mentally? Broke, stuck, trapped? These are temporary mental constructs or states of mind.

Mike Todd, a film producer in the 1950s, once said, "I've

never been poor, only broke. Being poor is a frame of mind. Being broke is a temporary situation." Mr. Todd made and lost several fortunes and was very careful to differentiate between a (potentially) permanent mental state and a temporary state of affairs. It is important for you to differentiate what your "why" may mean and if it is permanent or temporary. For example, is paying off your student loans your reason—or your "why"—for working at a painful but well-compensated job? If so, once the loans are paid off, you are definitely moving from this temporary why to a more permanent, meaningful why. If the reason you are working at your current job is that you must live close to your wife's family, then barring a large-scale migration of her family or divorce, your why is not changing and is most likely permanent.

Asking "why" can help determine what you want and need and where you are. Then it can provide a path for going forward. This is a critical step in the self-discovery and recovery process for you!

LOOK OUT ACROSS THE LAND

So what do you want? What do you need? Where do you want to be? How do you get that? And most importantly, why?

Those are seemingly innocuous questions, but they determine your life, work, mate, happiness, and future. Yet, those are the hardest questions to answer and may change over time.

What you need is what will bring emotional satisfaction

and happiness. Is it happiness, personal fulfillment, a strong, loving family? Those are pertinent, overarching needs. What you need is what you were placed on the earth to do. What you want typically is more material things, such as a new car or a fancy vacation.

The primary issue: What you need can be difficult to discern, difficult to accept, or difficult to do. Asking why moves the process forward.

Finding what you need and why takes reflection, soul searching, most likely some mistakes, loss, courage, and initiative. It is not easy.

Part of the reason we're asking these questions is to become more self-aware and explore those thoughts, needs, and feelings. If you were already more in touch with your feelings, you would've noticed you were getting burned out before it actually occurred and taken steps to correct it. You also would've been more in tune with whether you were doing what you actually want to do.

It took me a year of working less than full time, lots of reading, introspection, and thinking to get to the point of possibly knowing what I need and want to do and accomplish with my life. If your wants, needs, and desires are more aligned with your life and activities, there's much less risk for burnout.

FIND YOUR VALUES

Ask yourself some very basic, important, core value questions. Sit down, grab a writing implement and some paper, and actually answer these questions. If you (and I) can't get this right, all the steps after this will be in the wrong direction. If the overwhelming "why" is difficult to figure out, then the following questions may help you down the path of discovery.

- What did you do for fun when you were ten years old?
- What excites you?
- What activities do you "lose yourself" in for hours at a time? (I found myself writing for hours without realizing that time had passed.)
- What comes easily for you? Here's a hint: things that come naturally to you are your strengths. You may want to stop wasting time doing things that are difficult for you. There is a large body of thought in the American psyche and the American work ethic that tells us we should always strive to do the hardest things. In general, to combat burnout in the quickest fashion, you may want to go where your strengths are. This is what will come easily for you and will not frustrate you or not make your blood boil. Doing hard things can lead to more burnout or a slower recovery.

Write down your responses to the above questions. This will help you keep these thoughts organized. Put them on index cards if you like so you can regroup them into different areas and bundles as you organize and prioritize them in your mind. Give yourself time to do this.

Do any of the above answers have anything to do with what you do all day, every day to derive income or revenue? If not, you may not be in the right field.

Take a personality or strengths assessment (Kolbe, Clifton Strengths Finder). These may hold the hidden keys to what are your real talents, strengths, and desires.

BRING A NEW YOU INTO BEING

Once you have answered your questions and crystallized what you need and want, follow the next steps:

1. DECLARE WHAT YOU WANT AND NEED

Not "It would be nice" or "Someday, I'll get around to it." This declaration is a hell-bent-for-glory, not-taking-no-for-an-answer, get-out-of-my-way kind of declaration. This is the type of declaration that gets you off your backside, on your feet, reading, learning, and acting. Declaring what you want is deciding what your future will be. And yes, this can and will be scary. Courage is defined not as acting without fear but acting in the face of fear. Be courageous. Think about a time when you were scared of doing something, you did it, and in retrospect, the imagined fear you had was three to five times worse than the actual doing. Imagine this for yourself now.

The Latin root for "decide" is *decidere* or "to cut off." You are cutting off all other options. You are burning your boats after landing. There is no going back to the way you were or the life you had previously accepted. You are creating a life of your design, not of chance and occurrence. Now do I have your attention?

Essentially, reading this book is step one of hundreds and thousands until you get to where you want to be. This will be a process and a journey. It will take vision, commitment, and persistence. Author Stephen King received hundreds of rejection letters for his writing in his career. That did not dissuade him from continuing to write and submit his work. That is the dedication and single-minded focus that I want you to channel for your wants and needs.

You have to feel that passionate about your needs and wants. That is the fuel for you to make changes. Squishy goals lead to squishy or no results. Write down a declaration with a date. One of mine was, "I am going to finish this book no matter what!" Due date June 1, 2019. I got it done!

What would this look like for you? What do you want? For me, this want was fixing myself and my life no matter what it took. That ended up being the multifaceted exploration, journey, and set of actions that you will learn about throughout this book.

2. MANIFEST WHAT YOU WANT AND NEED

You have to love a word like "manifest" that is a noun, an adjective, and a verb. We are using the verb version of manifest: to make evident or certain by showing or displaying.

My personal definition of manifestation is bringing something into being that wasn't there before. You are creating a new reality and life for yourself. That is something that was not there before. You are bringing a new "you" into being. I am not trying to be melodramatic here, but nothing short of your conceptualizing this new "you" will bring about the changes you desire.

Once you find what you need, ignore the noise around you. Structure your life to get what you want and need. This takes doing, effort, guts, and gumption.

The doing is the scary part. That means you are actually committed to moving in a new direction, one that is not the same as the last one, five, ten, or more years of your life. And with commitment, there is action. Action will move you in the new, correct direction. This direction may be 180 degrees from where you were headed previously.

For example, what I need is to teach and to bring value to others with my contributions. How I am now doing that involves restructuring my life to include time for writing, speaking at community, state, and national events, running a support group, and offering my expertise when and where possible. Taking new action has been scary and adrenergic, but it feels right and good.

The only way this works is if you believe in what you need and want, where you want to go, and that you are worth it. You must believe that you are worth the time, effort, money, and energy to make changes.

I tell my vasectomy consult patients, "You wouldn't be sitting here if you weren't already 99 percent sure of your decision." The same goes for you. You wouldn't be sitting here (or reading this) if you weren't already 99 percent sure of your decision, which is to do something and change your life. If you do not, no one else will. The real questions are why and how. I do not ask my vasectomy patients to do their own vasectomies. That is why they come to see me. I similarly will not ask you to know exactly how to get to where you want to be. That is why you are reading this book.

HOW TO CHANGE: LOVE YOURSELF

How do you believe in yourself and your ability to change? The quickest way I have found to believe in yourself and make changes is to love yourself. In Kamal Ravikant's book, *Love Yourself Like Your Life Depends on It*, he details his process. Below is my interpretation of his work. The reason we need to relearn to love ourselves is that as physicians, we rarely think we are good enough and worthy of love, especially from ourselves.

In this exercise and definition of loving yourself, we are not talking about love in the egotistical, smarmy, kiss-my-own-biceps kind of way. This is love in the kind, forgiving, taking-all-of-your-good-and-bad, accepting kind of way. You are worth it. You are worth fighting for. The process is straightforward, and you can start right now. This is entirely how simple it is:

Tell yourself: "I love myself" truly, honestly, deeply, right now, fifty times.

Go ahead. I'll wait. This can be silent or out loud. Out loud is better, as research shows the sound reinforces what your mind is hearing and believing. Close your eyes if you like. Feel the power of those words. You don't necessarily even need to believe it right away. We are creating new thought patterns.

As hard as most physicians are on themselves, loving

yourself in this way will be a paradigm shift. The seven to fifteen years of training between medical school and residency have beaten an unhealthy sense of self-doubt, loathing, and loss of self-confidence into most physicians.

The process takes time, repetition, intention, energy, focus, and forgiveness if you stray while doing the phrase. Refocus if you get off track and keep repeating "I love myself, I love myself, I love myself." Do it while you are walking. Do it while you are ordering a latte. Do it before you go to bed. There is no limit to how much you can or should do this practice.

OK, who feels different? How? Better? Lighter? More relaxed? Hopeful? I always see improvement in myself after doing this exercise. Feel free to repeat your self-love ritual daily or multiple times a day. The bottom line is this: Love yourself enough to do this and to make changes.

As you think about your mental process for making change, think about going toward something you want, and not away from something you don't want. Avoidance of bad-ness is important and potentially lifesaving. But you are now not going to merely accept avoidance of badness. That would be like more resiliency training. I am calling BS on that. Let's get you thinking and moving toward what you want and need and the new you! In defining your "why," focus on what you are moving toward will get your mental picture to match what you are creating. You are building a bridge to cross the chasm from here to your future self. Do not perish regarding your vision! It is your guidepost forward. It is a critical component in determining your direction and where you want to go and, most importantly, beginning your recovery from burnout.

CHAPTER 6 TAKEAWAYS

- Your "why" takes effort and exploration to define.
- Your "why" drives your priorities in life.
- Question yourself regarding what you need, want, and why.
- Declare and manifest what you need.
- It will take action and be scary!
- You are worth it.
- Love yourself.

CHAPTER 7

Habits

How to Get There!

"We first make our habits, then our habits make us."

—JOHN DRYDEN

How in the world do you actually make change? How do you attack your burnout? I am trying not to leave you in the middle of the lake with no paddle. First, you need a plan, as you are outlining above and below. Then what? You are where you are because of the results of your actions. What determines your actions? To a large extent, your habits do. Studies show that up to 40 percent of our actions throughout the day are determined by habits, or reflexive automatic behaviors.[56] Habits help us navigate life without being overwhelmed by stimulation, which completely drains our mental energy and attention. What determines change? Your habits determine your behavior, which determine your ability to change. Your ability to alter your habits and form new ones leads to change.

What is useful about habits? Habits eliminate conscious

---

56 David T. Neal, Wendy Wood, and Jeffrey M. Quinn, "Habits—A Repeat Performance," *Current Directions in Psychological Science* 15, no. 4 (2006): 198–202.

choices, mostly negative choices, such as "I will eat bad food" or "I will stay in bed for another hour and not go to the gym." Those are useful habits, as they narrow the possibility of behaviors to ones that are beneficial to you, such as better nutrition and fitness. By eliminating conscious choice with the rote behavior of habit, we avoid opportunity to misbehave. I know that if we have Oreos (which are delicious) in our house, I will eat at least twenty of them. At seventy calories per Oreo, that is more than one-third pound of calories in Oreos. If there are no Oreos in my house, I will never buy, eat, or think about them. One-third pound of calories saved! The habit for me is not buying them.

Habits may also make you continue behaviors that are harmful, such as staying in a job that is killing your soul. Those are important life choices that have become hijacked by habit. Newton's first law of motion states, there is a "tendency of an object in motion to remain in motion." Newsflash: You are the object. You will tend to remain in your current motion, good, bad, or ugly, unless you make a change. This is why we are focusing on habit change. Once you are set in new, positive, productive habits or motions, you can start thinking about choice again within the realm of positivity, not negativity.

WHAT IS A HABIT REALLY?

A habit is a cue, a behavior, and a reward. Charles Duhigg, a Pulitzer Prize-winning journalist and author of *The Power of Habit*, details the extent to which habits control our lives and how we can turn the tables on them to take back control. For habit change to occur, the simplest series of events to facilitate change is leaving the cue, or trigger, for a behavior the same, as well as the reward for your behavior, but insert a new behavior. Some people bite their nails as a method of stress release. The cue is stress. The reward is stress release and a feeling of control. The behavior is nail biting. What if the behavior was humming your favorite song? The cue could be a stressful event, the behavior would be a rousing, hummed rendition of "Take Me Home" by Phil Collins, but the reward would still be feeling better as it is your favorite song. A bad habit is now changed, and manicure expenditures go way down!

KEYSTONE HABITS

A critical component of habit change is identifying and acting on changing keystone habits. Keystone habits are different for each person, such as quitting smoking for a smoker or learning new responses to unexpected, irritating events for me. Changing a primary habit causes a cascade of other positive habit changes once the change process is learned and internalized. For example, the smoker quits smoking, takes what they have learned from that behavior change success, then starts exercising, eats better, loses weight, becomes a responsible, reliable worker, learns to invest his or her money, and has positive, increasing results.

The process of habit change, in a nutshell, from Duhigg's classic text[57] is:

1. Change one keystone habit that you can control.

---

57 Charles Duhigg, *The Power of Habit: Why We Do What We Do in Life and Business* (New York: Random House, 2012).

2. Have a goal in your life! Habits love the motivation of a goal.
3. To change a habit, you must keep the old cue and deliver the old reward but insert a new routine, as explained above and below.
4. Belief accelerates and improves habit change, and belief happens easier when it occurs within a community.
5. A community provides support, and support happens best in groups.
6. Small wins lead to keystone habit change, which encourages other changes by creating structures that help other habits to flourish.
7. Willpower is the single most important keystone habit for individual success, and willpower itself becomes a habit by choosing a certain behavior ahead of time and then following a routine when opportunities for failure appear.
8. Control/autonomy. Research shows that willpower (number seven above) is even more effective when the sense of control people had over their experience was perceived as high.

For personal change, the preceding eight points are the path forward. Institutions also have habits, and not surprisingly, those can change as well. Data shows that on an institutional basis, increasing worker autonomy increased productivity[58] and reduced stress and stress-related health consequences.[59] These are all habits that can be implemented. Toyota Motor Corporation has long-standing,

---

58 C. O. Longenecker, J. A. Scazzero, and T. T. Standfield, "Quality Improvement through Team Goal Setting, Feedback, and Problem Solving: A Field Experiment," *International Journal of Quality and Reliability Management* 11, no. 4 (1994): 45–52.

59 *The Wall Street Journal*, March 2–3, 2019, p. C3.

strong support of the worker habit to stop the assembly line if even one worker perceives a problem. In the short term, productivity was lower, but by finding and fixing errors incrementally, giant productivity and quality improvements were seen. This is a productive, institutional keystone habit.

For large-scale institutional change, keystone habits drive change by aligning habits with corporate culture such that priorities are maintained, even when under duress.

To reduce burnout on an institutional level, physician wellness must become a keystone institutional habit, focus, and priority. I hope this book becomes a mechanism to drive that change. However, change, even on an institutional level, would multiply faster if it can be spread. According to Duhigg, for new keystone habits "to grow beyond a community, [they] must become self-propelling. And the surest way to achieve that is to give people new habits that help them figure out where to go on their own."[60] We hope and pray that physician wellness, care, and change become the new medical institutional keystone habit.

HABIT CHANGE

For habit change to occur, you must decide to change it. Once you have decided and cut off all other possibilities, you must identify the cues and rewards of your habits. Find alternative, productive behaviors. You have the control and awareness to accomplish this. Now that you know habits can change, you have the power and duty to act.

---

60 Duhigg, *The Power of Habit*, 239.

Habits can then be used for your benefit. All that is left is the doing. The process of habit change is powerful. Choose to change your problematic habits now. Then Newton's first law of motion about inertia is on your side, pushing you toward new habits and your goals automatically, by habit.

For your process, describe a problematic habit:

- What is the cue? Is it a person, a certain set of circumstances, a recurrent scheduling problem?
- What is the behavior? Do you become angry, frustrated, do something harmful or nonproductive?
- What is the reward? Do you have release of anger or stress, a feeling of "being right," a sense of control?

Let's walk through some habit change for you. Think of some part of your burnout, which could be a keystone habit, or something that just makes your blood boil. Usually, that would be the same thing. For me, if I had to pinpoint one damaging keystone habit, it would be a strong link between my ego and productivity. Breaking that link was the habit I needed to change. I was constantly checking the group and my personal productivity, which led to stress, anxiety, and frustration when I was not our most productive physician. I was focusing on productivity, what the components were, rearranging my practice to maximize that productivity, and feeling satisfaction when that occurred and frustration when it did not. The cue was our daily productivity report, the behavior was checking it multiple times a day, and the reward was satisfaction or frustration based on the data in the report.

By changing that keystone habit to checking the productivity report once a month instead of multiple times a day, I started to work less, took better care of myself, and wrote this book. Once I broke the link between happiness/frustration and productivity, I became much more focused on goals for my group and long-term strategic projects. Our productivity and success actually increased by letting go of the narrow focus on myself.

Consider possible keystone habits for you in your treatment of burnout. Remember that we are trying to change bad habits. Below are examples of bad professional habits:

- Reacting to negative situations with frustration and anger first.
- Physician wellness is the lowest priority.
- Valuing yourself last.
- Provider mental health is not a priority of the medical establishment.
- Bad or nonexistent mental health care is OK for physicians.
- Or something of equal importance to you.

You decide what is your keystone habit. That very directly informs and organizes all your personal and institutional behavior around the formation, honoring, and actions for that habit.

If you are not sure what your keystone habit is, start with just about any other undesirable habit you wish to change. This will show you the process and give you a small win. Then you can apply what you learned to your keystone habit.

Recognize what your cue or trigger is, insert a new behavior, and let the reward remain as is. Sounds simple, right? Well, as we say, recognizing that you have a problem is the first step. Developing a system for recognizing the cue is a key first step. If possible, keep track of trigger events, either on paper or in your phone. See how many cues you get in a day or week. That's all you have to do at first—to notice what your cue is. What might you notice right before your response? Frustration, anxiety, a physical sensation? Heat, mental confusion, a twitch? For me, I could definitely feel heat in my head and my blood pressure rising. Once you notice your cue, note it, then try to replace your subsequent behavior with a different behavior—for example, saying "Oh boy" or "That's neat"—or a physical act such as taking five or ten deep breaths. Then get your reward. Typically, that may be some sort of release of pent-up emotion, mental relief, or physical relaxation.

Think of the cue-behavior-reward cycle of a drug addict. There is an initiating event, such as stress or frustration. The typical response to the stress is drug use to get the reward of relieving that stress or frustration, at least temporarily. So the giant success of support groups like Narcotics Anonymous is replacing the behavior (drug use) with speaking with a sponsor or going to a support group. The cue is the same: stress. The reward is the same: feeling better. The behavior is the difference: productive conversation instead of destructive substance use.

In my own process, I took the cue to my stress—the report about my productivity—and changed the behavior to checking it only once a month instead of multiple times a day. That way, I got the reward of satisfaction without having the stress of the daily ups and downs in my productivity. My frustration around this behavior completely disappeared. My stress went down by 50 percent. But it still took me months to realize how critical this behavior change was to my overall mental and physical health. This was my keystone behavior.

The best solutions for constructing new habits and a new life are going to be the ones you make for yourself. They will be the most powerful because they are habits of your own design and the new habits you are developing. They will mean the most to you because they are yours. You are aligned intellectually, emotionally, and personally with your own solutions. Our philosophy for change is helping you to find your own solutions. They will resonate and empower you.

You may feel overwhelmed or that you do not know where to start. Changing habits requires significant mental, physical, emotional, and awareness capital to succeed. When faced with such a potentially daunting task, I can hear good ol' Eleanor Roosevelt in my head, encouraging me to move forward: "You must do the thing you think you cannot do."

It is surprising how easily what I thought I could not do becomes doable after moving past limiting thoughts. Habit change is key to making progress to burnout treatment. Start anywhere and do what you think you cannot! Let's get ready to take action! Forming great habits will then allow you to form yourself greatly. And having good habits will equip you with two paddles so you are not rowing around your lake in circles. You will then be ready to attack your burnout and reframe your life by taking action and build a new one. To begin this process, we reconstruct the component parts of your life, also known as "Your Box"!

CHAPTER 7 TAKEAWAYS

- Habits determine your behavior, which determines your results.
- Cue. Behavior. Reward.
- Attacking keystone habits leads to major change.
- Habit change is a learned process, which can be taught and repeated.
- Promoting physician wellness must be a keystone habit to drive healthcare system change.
- Practice on yourself by noticing your cues, replacing negative action with positive action, and getting your reward!
- Do what you think you cannot!

PART III

Action

CHAPTER 8

Life Construction

What Is a Box? What Is Your Box?

"The box that I've built around me is equal to the fear that is within me."

—CRAIG D. LOUNSBROUGH

An impolite use of the word *box* medically, as a verb, means for a patient to die, or end up in a box in the ground, as in "the patient boxed." My use of the word *box* describes life situations. If a person's personal box of their life construction is tight, constraining, frustrating, or limiting enough, it could lead to a literal box in the ground for that person, either from stress, burnout, secondary disease, or suicide. I am not saying that your box contains only fear, as Craig Lounsbrough might suggest. Your box contains your whole life, including your burnout. Little bits of burnout, or what has led you to burnout, are incorporated into every part of your life box.

That frustration you feel with your call schedule and its demands on you is part of the work environment wall of your box. The poor-quality, insufficient sleep you get while on call is part of your physical wall. The financial arrangements of your life that leave you feeling trapped are woven into your financial wall. There are multiple components of every wall of your burnout box that can and deserve to be fixed. Making the necessary changes and repairs to your box is the path to recovery from burnout. Let's define your box and show you how to deconstruct and rebuild a new one before you end up trapped in your current box in the ground.

Like any box, yours consists of a floor, walls, and a ceiling. They are there because those structures give a framework, support, direction, and protection to your life. That is important, and how you got where you are. But at this point, they may be limiting and harming you and your life. Assessing what you have wall by wall, component by component, will create a new, better box and a better structure to define, correct, and direct your life.

The box components are the floor, or your personal baseline. This is the sum total of all of your life experience, education, and previous beliefs.

The sides are:

- Work environment wall, which comprises the structure, tasks, pay, and responsibilities of your occupation.
- Mental wall is the sum of your mental models, paradigms, and thought processes.
- Physical wall consists of your health, nutrition, fitness, and sleep.
- Financial wall contains your attitudes and ideas about money, spending, creating value, and options.

- Spiritual wall holds your spirituality, faith, and belief in a Higher Power.
- Social wall is your relationship with others and the positive or negative interactions that can occur.
- The ceiling of the box represents any limits or beliefs you may have about yourself and your life.

With these definitions, let's reconstruct a new box for you!

A NOTE ABOUT ACTION

You are where you are as a result of your actions or inactions. Start somewhere with something. Actions that you take are all additive and accretive. They build on each other. And they become addictive but in a good way. Once you see progress from one action, the next one is easier because your mind already sees the previous success.

Combating burnout and changing your outcomes and life are *daily* practices. They require commitment. But you are really only trying to save your career and life. Isn't that worth a daily commitment? Of course it is. *IT* IS WORTHWHILE. We are talking about YOUR LIFE!

Improving yourself makes for better decision making, which then makes you feel and perform better, which then improves your decision making. This is a positive, never-ending, upward spiral. This process is something that will take work, effort, and commitment. It may take weeks to months to outline where you are for all of your walls, floor, and ceiling. Then it may take weeks to months to make the changes to get you moving in the right direction. That is OK! This is a marathon, not a sprint. And what could be more important than aligning your priorities and goals with your life? The surprising little side benefit of this process is that your burnout will get better. It may not completely go away, but your life box construction will be so much improved that burnout will become a much smaller, more manageable part of your life. If and when it rears its ugly head again, you are already equipped to assess, manage, and fix it with this process. By no means do we want you to "box"! Your new box will contain not only fear but also your new life. Let's explore the parts of your box, starting with your floor.

CHAPTER 8 TAKEAWAYS

- Your box is your life, burnout and all!
- Action determines results.
- Combating burnout is a daily practice.
- Don't "box"! Fix your box! Treat your burnout!

CHAPTER 9

Your Floor

"If no one ever took risks, Michelangelo would have painted the Sistine floor."

—NEIL SIMON

The real risk for you is not examining what provides the foundation for your life: your floor. The floor of your box is the sum of all your past experiences, education, and life learning. This also contains all of your subconscious input and learning over your entire life, both positive and negative. It includes any trauma. Your floor is where you stand, literally and figuratively. For me, this includes previous erroneous thoughts such as "Money is bad," horrible experiences such as my brother's carjacking and murder, and my historical responses to frustration. Your floor issues can be significant. These issues contribute to burnout and may not let you change or adapt to treat your burnout unless you handle them. You may need to simultaneously attack some of your floor issues while acting on the walls and ceiling of your box. This may include counseling, medical therapy, tears, anguish, and change. Please seek all the care you need for yourself and your "floor" issues.

The process for assessment, planning, and action for the

floor, walls, and ceiling is similar as far as how to start, make changes, and implement a plan.

Take a piece of paper, or three Excel spreadsheets, three notepad documents from your iPad, chalk and chalkboard, or a hunk of coal, and your wall. Whatever works for you is best. Divide the space or documents into three sections. List what you have/where you are now on the left, and what you want/where you are going on the right.

Leave the middle blank for now. The middle section is for your action steps. It can be one step for going through your process on the left to something on the right, or it can be many. A step can be large or microscopic. That is 100 percent up to you. Some people like to cross off many action steps. Others like to cross off only giant chunks of accomplishment. Whatever works for you is best.

This process can be daunting. Sometimes it is easier to start closer to your goal/declaration and work backward to where you are now. What would be the last step before your goal, and the next previous, then the next previous, until you arrive to where you are now and have what you have now. Chunk it back from the end. Making a giant mental leap from left to right may never be possible. Sometimes it may make more sense for you to inch forward. Taking small, achievable steps, either forward or backward, will get you there.

For example, let's say you want to move on from something foundational in your personal history in the floor portion of your box, such as "Money is bad" for me. I think that thought construct came from the mentality growing up in

Iowa that you really didn't show off your money, and if you did, you were being boastful. That, in my mind, became "Money is bad." The end thought for me is, "Money is a tool."

WHERE YOU ARE/ CURRENT THOUGHTS	ACTION STEPS	WHERE YOU WANT TO GO/NEW THOUGHTS
Money is bad.	Money experiences and emotions	
	Hanging out with money	
	Net worth?	
	I have money and I am not bad.	
	Money use list	Money is a tool.

The first step from the left side was recounting my experiences with money and messages I had perceived that led to this false thought pattern. I had heard or inferred that as I was growing up we may have not had a lot of money but were doing something important, as both of my parents were educators. As an adult, I evaluated that belief with an adult mind, objectively determining its validity. After this assessment, I came to the realization that money, education, and the utility of money are all important. The next step was hanging out with money, having discussions about the utility of money, seeing how other people used and dealt with money. The following step was taking a calculator to my assets and liabilities to figure my net worth and discovering that it was greater than zero. I am not sure what "rich" is, but I have never felt that way. The next step just was realizing that I had some money, but I was not bad. That is a tough subject and took some convincing of myself.

The final step was making a list of all the uses of money and listing "Good" or "Bad" next to them. More than 90 percent of my list was "Good." Therefore, money is a tool, not inherently good or bad.

Now I have deconstructed that thought process for you. But in order to fully process it and make that change, realize how those thoughts make you feel. You may get anxious, angry, and self-righteous about that thought. The emotion previously associated with your thought about "bad money" was a stressor and caused some unhealthy behaviors in your life, most likely self-sabotage, making poor financial decisions to keep you from getting money and therefore becoming "bad" in your own mind. Take the same energy of emotion but direct it toward the contrapositive. Literally, think "Money is good" and feel what that is like. Bless it. Feel positivity toward money and people who have money. Money will not come to you if you have negative thought patterns about it.

You are creating a new thought pattern, a new groove in your brain, a new habit, and a new response. It will take practice and self-awareness, and you must catch yourself when you see the old way of thinking, stop it, and repeat the positive emotion. You have a lifetime of positive and negative experiences that make up your floor. Get the negative thoughts and beliefs identified and realigned. Become the Michelangelo of your life, take the risk, and paint your own Sistine Chapel, floor to ceiling! It will be worth it. Once some of your life foundation floor issues are tackled or improving, you will have firm ground to start working on your walls and recovery from burnout.

CHAPTER 9 TAKEAWAYS

- Your floor is the sum of your life experiences and learning.
- Define and rebuild your floor issues in the three-panel process.
- Create new thought patterns to redefine your floor.

CHAPTER 10

─────

Your Work Environment Wall

"I like work: it fascinates me. I can sit and look at it for hours."

—JEROME K. JEROME

If you are like more than 90 percent of physicians, your work environment may be a significant or even the sole source of your burnout.[61] Unlike Mr. Jerome, for the typical physician, there is not much sitting around. You always seem to have plenty of work to do. As a urologist, I get five or more job offers a day from around the country. I never have to worry about having a job. It's whether I can thrive in my work environment. Hence, this book is designed to help you thrive. I like to break down what determines your work environment in the simplest of terms.

For most jobs, it boils down to:

1. What you give.
2. What you get.
3. How do you get out.

─────

61 Jeff Moody, personal research, 2019.

What you give to medicine may include your licensing and training, your intelligence, your work ethic, your time, your billing expertise, your diligence, your empathy, your compassion, your nighttime hours, your weekend hours, the possibility of contracting an infectious or deadly disease, the possibility of being sued or shot by a patient, your marriage, your relationships with important people in your life, your patience, your leadership, your blood, your health, your soul, and your life. Whew! What a list! Did anyone ever think signing on to this job was akin to a deal with the devil?

What you get can include the unbelievable satisfaction and joy of helping another human being in a small or a lifesaving way, income, prestige, status, investment opportunities, stress, ulcers, fabulously poor health, free lunch or no lunch, sleep deprivation, a crash course in business, an on-the-job MBA with variable results, management and marketing education, a crash course in how to use an Excel spreadsheet to calculate your compensation or lack thereof, a divorce, suicidal ideation, and of course, BURNOUT. Right off the bat, I am not sure what any of us get as physicians is worth what we give.

How you get out can include working for more than thirty years and retiring, "slowing down" and moving to a part-time track, becoming employed versus owning, exiting clinical medicine and working in medically related fields, leaving medicine entirely and choosing a new career, locum tenens, suicide, or what most physicians do and what I like to call the slow burn. This is when you are trapped in a work/compensation environment partially of your creation or acceptance, hate it, but now would require blowing up your entire life to change it, or so you think.

Let's tilt the scales in our favor. You have more control, discretion, and influence over your environments than you think.

There are a number of different scales or levels of work environments. I like to break it down into three: macro-, mecro-, micro-environments.

Your macro work environment includes your life as a doctor, the overall economy, the Centers for Medicare and Medicaid Services and their rules and regulations, and the hospital or health system in which you work. We have relatively limited influence on our macro-environment. If you don't like it, you could move to another country. Life is full of choices.

The micro-environment is the day-to-day, desktop, office, or operating room work construct within which you perform your job. The decision cake here may already be baked, meaning what and how you do may already be decided by the work setting or business entity you are joining. This does not mean this micro-environment cannot be changed or improved but that it may take time or may not be possible.

Be careful who you join, and be fully aware of how the micro-environment works or doesn't. Always get any promises of work environment structure made to you in writing. A large number of my friends have taken jobs with health systems, were promised many things, started working, and then the promises changed. Surprisingly, the changes never seem to be in the new employee's favor. "Hey, sorry, we are going to have to double your salary and cut your call in half." Nope, that never happens. Uniformly, the deal gets worse. You have now jumped ship to this new job and cannot easily go back. Get your promises in writing.

If your micro-environment EMR is indeed driving you batty, I have several suggestions. First, get a swipe card for logging on, rather than typing a username/password. This will save thousands of keystrokes a year. Second, as a HealthPartners Minneapolis study showed, using standardized workflows and teams, collaborative and streamlined documentation and in-basket management[62] saves one hour and fifteen minutes a day. Third, a scribe or medical transcriptionist working at your side will remove 90 percent of your headaches in dealing with your EMR. We use a modified scribe system in my practice with very good results. And the cost is usually less than one extra patient per day. The benefits are nearly immeasurable! It is possible to slay the EMR beast! I do have to thank my EMR for two things, though. It got me thinking about how I want to practice medicine. Also, my EMR actually took away any spare time I had, so it radically decreased my online shopping, and it may actually be a break-even deal for the cost of the EMR versus what I was spending online.

In between macro and micro is the mecro work environment, which is my own made-up word for the workspace between macro and micro to describe not global and not desktop decisions, and environments, and because "e" is between "a" and "i." (Meso is probably the right prefix, but it sounds boring and doesn't phonically fit with the other

---

62 A.-M. Audet et al., "Information Technologies: When Will They Make It into Physicians' Black Bags?" *MedGenMed* 6, no. 4 (2004): 2.

two. Plus, I always wanted to make up a word, and it's my book, so my word. If you want to make up a word, write your own book!)

Mecro work environment describes the intermediate space where the decisions that guide and control our lives occur, such as what job to take, what you are paid, how much call you take, and where to live. These are the box-constructing decisions. These are the agreements that you have made with others and yourself. Your control of your mecro work environment will govern a large part of your happiness, work satisfaction, and potential for burnout.

How do you control your mecro-environment? By knowing yourself, what makes you happy and fulfilled at work, and how you work best. You must revisit what can go into your bullshit bucket. Remember, this is the container of all the aspects of your life that you tolerate but don't love. Only you can determine how full it can be and when you need to make changes in your work environment. Certainly, there are tradeoffs that can be made: "I will be on call for the weekend, but I get to take Monday off"; "I will cover the remote clinic three hours from my house, but we have a professional services agreement with the clinic, and I am paid separately and well for my efforts. Plus, I am providing care for a medically underserved area."

Think, anticipate, and design your mecro-environment to your own satisfaction. Do this at the outset of a job or actively work to improve the job parameters until they reach an acceptable benefits-bullshit ratio for you, which is completely subjective and up to your definition. I use my gastrointestinal barometer, or "gut," to determine my

B-B ratio. Ideally, the ratio should be over three to five or higher. You can be quite happy in that environment. If the ratio falls below one and is not fixable, it is time to consider a new work environment entirely or blow up the framework of your agreement and construct a new one.

In order to properly align your mecro-environment, you may want to ask yourself:

- What am I worth?
- What do my peers with similar experience, training, and skills command as pay?
- What do I add that is above and beyond that skillset? What is that worth?
- What are my priorities?
- What income do I want to make?
- What hours do I want to work?
- Am I on call? How often? How onerous? Paid outside of my base pay?
- Do I have nonclinical responsibilities?
- Am I compensated for those responsibilities in time, money, or help?
- Do I have management or business responsibilities?
- Am I compensated for those responsibilities in time, money, or help?
- Does my compensation cover living expenses where I work?
- Is my compensation fixed, variable, or effort/RVU based?
- Am I paid on a pure production basis?
- Are there clinical and patient factors on which I am evaluated/paid?
- Benefits?

- Vacation?
- Continuing medical education?
- Opportunities or requirements to teach?
- Ownership or outside investment opportunities?
- Is there help (administrative, medical assistant, scribe, PA/NP) to decrease the irritating, time-sucking, burnout-inducing parts of your job?
- What EMR is used and how does it perform?
- Tell me about your Physician Wellness Program.
- If I am overburdened, when I take a new task or responsibility, I will drop an old one.
- I can trade time for money: I reserve the right to hire a scribe, change or drop insurance plans, drop Medicare, and generally say no to abusive demands!

Bottom line: Think, anticipate, and design your mecro-environment to your own satisfaction. If the current job you have under consideration does not fit, move on. Generally, it is very difficult for you to change a job or work environment from the outside as a new hire unless the organization has a history of extreme flexibility in job design for new hires.

By asking yourself the important questions above, you will be automatically setting yourself up to be successful, happy, and productive. And you will either go a long way in preventing burnout or changing your current work environment with burnout into one in which you control the potential to burnout.

Remember, control your work environment. Don't just "watch your work" as Mr. Jerome would say. Make your own decisions, or most certainly, someone else will make those decisions for you. Somehow, those decisions never seem to be to your benefit. Let's explore what may be driving some of your decisions: your mental wall.

CHAPTER 10 TAKEAWAYS

- Your work environment is a gigantic determinant of your burnout.
- What do you give and get, and how do you exit from your work?
- Control your work environments, macro, mecro, and micro.
- Slay your EMR beast with standardization, technology, tools, and scribes.
- Design and control the box-constructing agreements of your work environment.
- Calculate your benefit-bullshit ratio. Know your limits.
- Ask the right questions *before* accepting a work environment.
- Get the answers in *writing*.
- Treat the number one source of burnout: your work environment.

CHAPTER 11

Your Mental Wall

"Ideas that require people to reorganize their picture of the world provoke hostility."

—JAMES GLEICK

YOUR PARADIGMS

A new idea in your life may indeed provoke hostility within yourself. Perhaps more than any other wall, your mental wall is the lens through which you see the world. It is your framework and paradigm that governs your interpretation of what has happened in your life and what you have learned. It is a part of your past. Your mental wall paradigms also determine, more importantly, how you respond and what you do next. They lead to your future.

What are your paradigms? What are your guiding principles? What are your central tenets and beliefs? What are the things that guide how you live your life on a daily basis and control the decisions you make? How do they translate into your central plan but not like the five-year plans of the former Soviet Union? (We all know how well those worked out.)

Are some of them:

- Retire by sixty? Fifty? Forty?
- Make X number of dollars per year?
- Make more dollars than your sibling? Parent? Your "frenemy" from medical school?
- Have X amount of dollars in the bank by Y age?
- Become chair of the department?
- Be world renowned?
- Have X car or live in Y house in Z neighborhood?
- No one is going to screw me in a negotiation or a deal?

Can you see how the framework you set up for yourself, your guiding principles, will then determine every part of how you construct the rest of your life? Again, I am not saying that paradigms are not useful, but carried to an extreme or not adapted in a changing situation, those same paradigms become constricting, harmful, and boxlike.

For example, let's say I have a paradigm that says I will make X dollars per year. The current market rate for compensation for my specialty is X minus 20 percent. So what does my paradigm tell me? Work harder, take a second job, make potentially risky investments, all to make up the 20 percent. What is the toll, or blowback, from the sacrifices made to get that final 20 percent? Less free time as you work more, poorer health, poorer relationships, bad parenting of your kids, actual loss of money if your investments go bad? And that is just a very short list. The downstream effects can be lifelong and damaging. And why? All because you have a paradigm that is driving decision making that is ultimately harmful to you.

I am not going to say that your previous paradigms were unsuccessful. Whatever they were or are, they did get you to where you are now. You did, after all, pursue and complete a successful educational path through medical school and residency.

One of the main paradigms I was wedded to pre-burnout (and one that probably contributed mightily to my burnout) was that I was the most productive partner, saw the most patients, did the most work RVUs, and brought in the most money. Why? I think it had much to do with linking my self-worth to my productivity worth. It also made me feel that I was contributing to our group. In addition, I did most of the strategic management functions, acted as our junior banker, and was chief cook and bottle washer. I think my central tenet driving that construct was that we had to maximize our practice, and if I could help to do that, then I would. I forgot that I could actually ask for or hire help for those tasks.

However, the paradigms that worked when we were five, ten, twenty-five, or thirty-five years old may not work now. Life is a series of evolutions, and yet we stubbornly hold on to previous paradigms, or interpretive filters, that then determine our response or behavior patterns. We do this because they worked in the past and we do not know any new ones. Luckily, we can fix the second part of that equation, which will then lead to a new paradigm working for you. So how can we know what our paradigms are? I thought you would never ask.

EVALUATION OF YOUR PARADIGMS

Let's peel your onion. You have layers of your mental paradigms. One of the most straightforward methods I have experienced to peel this onion is the 5 Whys Exercise. What is the 5 Whys Exercise? It is an iterative process first used in the Toyota Motor Corporation in the 1950s to improve manufacturing processes. But the process is useful for getting to the center of your onion, or paradigm, that is controlling your life.

Define the problem, or in this case define what you think is causing your burnout, from a mental, paradigmatic standpoint. For example, "I must work/am trapped in this job in this way and make X dollars." Then ask, "Why?"

WHY? "Because I went to school for all those years and took out all those loans, and I must use my training and pay back those loans."

WHY? "To be respected and valued."

WHY? "Because I grew up disadvantaged, was made fun of, and vowed never to feel that way again."

WHY? "Because I was made to feel inferior by my family and friends."

WHY? "Because no one in my family ever finished high school, and I have no one to help guide me through my life."

Aha! There is the core motivation. Solution: Find a mentor to help guide you to a better place, thought process, and life. Whew!

Beware, the 5 Whys can uncover some pretty deep, emotional, sometimes salty, fear-inducing thoughts. Be prepared to face some thoughts that you have never thought of and their consequences. It can be an emotional, unsettling process. If so, that means you are getting to the core of the problem. You may need some help interpreting or dealing with the responses that this brings up. Do not hesitate to seek professional counseling or therapy during this process or at any time through your transition. But do not let your fear or discomfort stop you. Fear means you are close to making a significant change. Fear and discomfort are mechanisms your mind uses to maintain the status quo. If the status quo was so awesome, you would not be reading this book or doing these exercises. You would not be burned out already. Use the new realizations to change your paradigms and your life.

The 5 Whys can be applied to any problem. Now you may be starting to have a grasp on your previous paradigms. You have many to deal with, peel back, examine, fix, and redefine. The 5 Whys process may take you a long time, as you could have dozens of old paradigms. Keep digging away at them. Anytime you feel stuck, frustrated, or angry, mark where you are and take a (short) break. Come back when the emotion attached to the paradigm has cooled a little. Examine what triggered the emotional response, what is the root cause, and what is a possible solution. If that solution does not work, try another one. This is an iterative process, usually, and not a giant, light bulb, thunderclap realization. So, again, take your time, but keep moving forward.

NEW MENTAL PARADIGMS?

I am not going to mandate or install any new paradigms, mostly because you need to figure out what is going to work for you. Any new paradigms you develop will mean much more and be more effective if you actually develop them. What I would like to do, and have you consider, is a new construct, or the 2 x 4 framing for your new mental wall, a paradigm of paradigms, so to speak.

Simon Sinek is a business consultant, trainer, and speaker, who developed what he calls the Golden Circle paradigm for leaders with influence on organizations.

The "Golden Circle" from Simon Sinek

WHY

HOW

WHAT

WHY. HOW. WHAT.

The concept is that everyone knows what they or their business does. We make shoes. We make cars. We are doctors and care for patients. Most people can even tell you how they do it. Our shoe production plants are in Ohio. Our car production plants operate in Tennessee. We see patients and do surgery for their diseases. Very few people can tell you why they do what they do. "Um, because that is the job I have," or "This is what my family has always done," or "I went to medical school, so now I am a doctor." Those are not extremely powerful whys.

When you work from the inside out, from your WHY, your entire paradigm shifts. Your global view of WHAT you do starts to come from a powerful WHY.

MY GOLDEN CIRCLE

For myself, as I thought about this, WHY I do what I do, as a urologist, became much clearer. I realized after all the school, training, and work experience, my WHY for what I do is this: I am a trusted advisor in a time of need for a patient. HOW I do this is by accurate assessment of a patient's problem, formulation of a plan, communicating to the patient what the plan is, and putting that plan into motion. WHAT I do is move that plan forward by prescribing medicine, doing surgery, or referring the patient on for appropriate next steps.

Ah, that is quite a paradigm shift. When I came at it from the trusted advisor starting point, my lens shifted. Now I do not see continuing medical education requirements as a mandated chore by some outside governing body. I see them as an opportunity to become a better advisor. I don't see multiple patient questions as slowing down my clinic but as a chance to help a frightened, vulnerable person understand what their situation is and how we are going to help them. I take the time during an annual appointment not to just check their pulse and refill medicines but to also discuss with and educate the patient about new dietary and exercise recommendations for their disease. My WHY as a trusted advisor gave me a new appreciation and framework for HOW and WHAT I do. I gave better advice and provided higher value for my patients.

The WHY/HOW/WHAT Golden Circle can be applied to all other aspects of your life as well. Use it in parenting. Use it as you interact with your friends, colleagues, and staff. Use it in your financial planning. When you come from a powerful, well-thought-out, personally meaningful WHY, all the other decisions and processes are easy, clear, and now seemingly obvious. You are welcome!

If your paradigmatic universe has not already been blown to pieces by what you have learned so far in this chapter, the next level of paradigm-ism will:

BE. DO. HAVE.

In the Western world, material accumulation now seems to be the benchmark for personal success. Having is a top priority. The paradigm is, "Have a lot, then you can Do lots of things, and then you will Be a success."

Why do most lottery winners go bankrupt? Because they have skipped all the way to the Having step, without the time and work of Being and Doing. They have no paradigm or developed framework that led to the Having. So whatever is poured into their life runs out the bottom like a sieve because there is no framework or "box" to catch it. It disappears quickly.

I would like to turn that on its head. The paradigm for most successful people is that they will Be the person that they envision in their mind as a success, they will Do the work that needs to be done to become that person, and entirely as a by-product of Being and Doing, they Have success.

Be. Do. Have.

Success and Having are results or products of a successful paradigm, not first steps. If you can visualize who you want to be, put in place how to do that, having the results will be easy, natural, and expected. Colin Powell, former chairman of the Joint Chiefs of Staff and US secretary of state, worked his way through college prior to joining the military. He always treated any job he had—such as working as a janitor while in school—as the most important job possible, performing it with the utmost effort, quality, and excellence. He was going to be the best janitor he possibly could be. He was being a chief of staff and doing the caliber of work to get there just a few years before he actually had the job. Success is a habit, and how you do anything is how you do everything. Be who you want to become. Do the work. Have the results.

Be. Do. Have. QED.

Finally, from a mental wall or mindset standpoint, if you

do not learn anything from this entire book or change any part of your life in a positive direction other than this next concept, I would be ecstatic if you incorporated this one paradigm into your life:

BE GRATEFUL

You may say, "How can solving all my problems be that easy? I can recover from burnout by saying thanks enough? Just be grateful? I am grateful. I say thanks to my office staff at least once a month...But I am still burned out like crazy." Being grateful refocuses your energy and direction toward accepting all that occurs in your life and your response to it.

But how grateful are you? Are you grateful for waking up in the morning? Are you thankful for every patient you see and every successful case you do? Are you effusive with your thanks to your family for putting up with you? Are you grateful to the point where you get immense peace from your gratitude and people around you start to become annoyed with how grateful you are? Then, and only then, you are getting close to the right amount of gratitude.

Let's explore exactly what gratitude is. It can be defined as a feeling of appreciation or thanks. While gratitude is something that you typically express to others ("Thanks for the ride"), the vast majority of gratitude can be you expressing gratitude to yourself: "I am grateful for my health and the opportunity to serve others." If you are anything like me, you are probably a little short on the gratitude selfies. Appreciate yourself and all you do. As physicians, we are constantly self-evaluating. Did my treatment work? Was my surgery a success for the patient? Am I going to be sued? Am I an idiot? That avalanche of negative self-talk can bury any hint of self-love and gratitude. Turn off the self-flagellation on a regular basis—at least daily. Try it! Once per day at least, give yourself room to appreciate what you have done. This can be done by the "I love myself" exercise or by simply meditating on the positive aspects of your life if only for five or ten minutes per day. Feel good about it! Feel good about yourself! Thank yourself! All right!

Gratitude has levels of achievement or appreciation. Now that you can thank yourself, let's expand the circle of gratitude. The next level is gratitude toward others. It can be as simple as acknowledgment of the existence of someone doing a small favor or service for you, such as holding a door or pressing the elevator button for your floor. It can be thanking your office and OR staff every day and every case (as I do) for their work and efforts. It can be gratitude to your spouse and family for their understanding and humor. It can be a simple phone call to your parents thanking them for all they have done for you. You decide, but demonstrate your gratitude to others.

The next level is gratitude to a Higher Power in whatever way is meaningful to you. This does two things: you get to feel connection to that Higher Power, Source Energy, or The Force, and you get to take a load off yourself and outsource some of the endless pressure you may be applying to yourself, thus reducing your burnout.

Last, at the highest level of gratitude, there is a Zen/Confucius/Jedi mind trick, a sort of up-is-down, left-is-right kind of gratitude for even bad things that happen to you. With action, there is consequence, sometimes positive and sometimes negative. "Win or learn" is a phrase I like to describe any action and consequence pair. If there is an action with an unfavorable outcome, yes, that stinks, but what did you learn? Where is the lesson of gratitude in the bad consequence? "I had a car breakdown but got to spend time with my kids, learning about their lives, while we waited for AAA." "I spent a year in a horrible job but learned everything I needed to make the next job my dream job."

Use your gratitude to appreciate the lessons you learn from perceived negative consequences. This is the Dalai Lama, kiss-your-enemy level of gratitude. When you can divorce the results and your emotional response to those results from the learning, then you have snatched the pebble from my hand. I can teach you no more. Go into the world, grasshopper. You have reached the highest level of gratitude.

I recently was having some hesitancy about my plans with this book and the transition from full-time clinician to writer or whatever my new career might be. I was feeling some anxiety that I was moving too slowly and that my medical career might be slowing down that transition. I wasn't going fast enough! I was slightly resentful and not very grateful.

Then I stopped to think how, every day, I had the privilege and honor of practicing medicine and that was a gift. I was grateful for that. And how every day I practiced medicine, it taught me the valuable lessons I am now sharing, and I was grateful for that. And how every day I practiced medicine, which provided the emotional, intellectual, and financial capital to write this book and possibly pursue a new career, and I was grateful for that. Then I was not stressed or anxious anymore. And that the progression of me through this process is necessary, useful, appropriate, and something for which I am thankful.

Spare yourself endless mental gymnastics with harmful paradigms. Instead, change your paradigms! Use the energy and stress from previous paradigms, redirected in a new positive direction. New ideas and new paradigms may provoke hostility, but that means you are on the right track. They will help reduce your burnout. You are now mentally fit. Does your body match?

CHAPTER 11 TAKEAWAYS

- Your mental paradigms are the lens through which you view and react to the world.
- 5 Whys will drill down to the core of your motivations.
- The Why/How/What paradigm will create a deeper, more meaningful source of definition in your work.
- Be what you want. Do the work. Have the results.
- Be grateful, from yourself to the Source of all things good and bad.
- Upgrading your paradigms improves your life and reduces your burnout.

CHAPTER 12

Your Physical Wall

"I'm so unfamiliar with the gym, I call it James!"

—ELLEN DEGENERES

Your body is a temple. Why does it feel like an urban renewal project gone horribly wrong? Has it been so long since you have been to the gym that you can't even call it James?

We have spent a lot of time in this book exploring the mental and conceptual basis for how we have become burned out and ways back to a healthy functioning life via mental exercises and restructuring your thinking. The primary support for burnout recovery and a great life is your physical body and health, how it is functioning and how you care for it. Poor health, diet, and physical status are, most likely, contributing to your burnout. You would not expect a sports car to win races using bad motor oil or a thoroughbred horse to run on no sleep, but that is what we expect of ourselves on a daily basis.

Unfortunately, garbage in equals garbage out for our lives, our bodies, and our health. The act of constructing a new physical wall, with a quality outlook and plan for your physical body, health, and nutrition may be the first time you actually take your own medicine and apply all that you learned in medical school, residency, and your career to yourself. Doctor, heal thyself! Here we go!

MEDICAL CONDITIONS

In no way is this book meant to be actual medical advice. Yes, I am a doctor, but I cannot speak to your specific medical conditions, and although you may feel you know me through this book, we do not have an established doctor-patient relationship. What we do have is information. You know what medical conditions you have, and if, like me, you have not been to see another doctor in "some time," get to the dang doctor and get evaluated. Let's see where we are starting and improve from there. Recently, my own "annual" appointment took me three years to get to.

A sure way to increase the effect of burnout on you is to ignore chronic conditions that you may have, such as diabetes, hypertension, obesity, depression, arthritis, and anything else. Nothing makes a bad day worse than feeling like crap even at baseline. I know, the last thing you want to do when you are feeling bad, beaten down, and exhausted is go to the doctor. I know you probably don't want to take meds that may have side effects you don't like, make you think you are a patient, and even, short term, worsen how you feel. It can definitely be a downward spiral. But please, take your meds if you need them. And then let's concentrate on improving your general health so much that maybe you can get off some of your meds.

GENERAL HEALTH
SLEEP

Let's start with the easiest act to reduce burnout and promote recovery. This is something that requires no effort at all and allows you to be lazy and just lie down: sleep. The World Health Organization recently classified sleep deprivation as harmful to your health as smoking. Getting enough sleep purely from a health standpoint is job one!

There are three aspects to sleep: getting enough, getting quality sleep, and getting insomnia handled. We are on call (most of us), have work commitments outside of normal hours, and these sometimes occur in the middle of the night. Emergencies and patient care issues cannot be planned. Hence, the word *emergency*. There is nothing as unique (or exhausting) as operating most of the night and then having a completely full clinic day the next day. That's certainly not a recipe for burnout, is it?

The warrior physician mentality is, "We will sleep when we are dead." Well, that actually may be true. Studies show a direct correlation between decreasing sleep and decreasing life expectancy. See, you will get to sleep when you are dead sooner because you will be dead sooner!

A vanishingly small percentage of people (like 0.6 percent) have a gene that allows a fully functioning life and person on four to five hours of sleep at night. Now, I know physicians like to think of themselves as in the top 1 percent of everything, especially academically, but not all physicians could possibly have won this genetic lottery.

So how much sleep is enough? I am going to go out on

a limb and put a number out there: seven hours. That is about the minimum that will get you to the point of increasing your health and decreasing your risk of death to baseline. Less than six hours of sleep statistically appears to be a real danger point. Actually, more than eight to nine hours of sleep also starts to increase your risk of mental illness, health issues, and death as well. So seven hours appears to be the Goldilocks amount: just right.

Sleep quality also appears to be very important. Getting the right amounts of REM and deep sleep have statistically beneficial effects on your health and life as well.

Timing of your sleep can get you more bang for your sleep buck as well. The time slot from ten in the evening to two in the morning appears to be the golden hours for sleep. More deep sleep occurs in that time than at any other point in the night. The more of that particular time that you can actually be sleeping, the more beneficial it is to you.

STRUCTURING YOUR SLEEP

Like most elements of your environment, your sleep environment is more under your control than you think. Think about how small changes can make large differences in your sleep quantity and quality.

Let's start with work. As one of the primary demands on our time—and for physicians, one that can significantly impact sleep—work can be never ending. Since sleep is required for living effectively and reducing burnout, strategically structuring and planning for your sleep is critical. How can you do this?

Here are some options.

Hire Help

Consider physician extenders, shift coverage, and per diem workers to cover especially the more onerous and/ or painful night hours. One physician group I know was taking all of their own night call, so every night two to three of their group of twenty were not sleeping due to the busy nature of the practice and the hospital workload. So they hired three full-time "night" physicians—people who were night owls already. Every one of the "day" physicians then got to sleep and work when it was best for them. It did cost each physician a moderately significant amount per year to hire these other night doctors, but as one of the partners put it to me, "If you could look at a job with our group with no night call ever, with this lower salary, would you take this job?" They have nearly a 100 percent acceptance rate of job offers to new physicians. And their quality of life has skyrocketed.

Consider Shift Work

Take the twenty-four-hour duties and divide the hours so one person is not covering for undue amounts of time, forgoing sleep. Perhaps a "night" doctor can be assigned from 6:00 p.m. to 6:00 a.m. and cover those hours for several weeks consecutively with no day duties. Studies do show the absolute worst sleep/health outcomes accrue to those workers who "swing," or change shifts from day to evening to night on a regular basis. So please avoid torturing yourself and damaging your health like that.

Outsource Duties

There are outsourced radiology image-reading services in Australia that are happy to read imaging studies during their day, which is night in the Western hemisphere, so everyone can sleep at appropriate times.

Drop or Change Responsibilities or Your Job Description

OB/GYNs can drop obstetrics, increasing their sleep by a quantum leap. One of my OB friends who did this told me he cannot believe the difference in his life, mental acuity, and energy, after not sleeping well for thirty years. Anesthesiologists can transition to working at surgery centers with no night or weekend duties. Any physician can limit the scope of their practice by disease state, patient age, or insurance. Many physicians are transitioning to a concierge model, charging an annual fee for caring for a patient on the doctor's panel, providing more personalized care (house calls, hospital rounding if the patient is admitted, accompanying patients to their other doctor appointments) and limiting their total patient load to 10 to 30 percent of the previous panel. This provides striking beneficial results for the concierge doctor's life and sleep.

Open Your Mind to the Options That Are Available to You

I know some of you may be employed physicians and feel that you do not have as much or any control over your environment or expenditures. If so, meet with your employer or hospital system and have a serious heart to heart about how beneficial it is keeping you, the engine of their system, happy, healthy, and well slept. And just let them know that replacing you, if you have health issues or just leave due to a poor work environment, will cost them between $500,000 and $1 million. And as we have discussed previously, studies have shown that physicians who are burning out are more likely to go to part-time work, reduce productivity, and provide poorer care with an increased rate of errors. Your employer will pay for lots of help for you to avoid those negative financial impacts. Also, your malpractice carrier certainly would like you to get enough sleep to prevent errors, patient harm, and lawsuits.

Sleep Environment

Your sleep environment can have an outsized impact on your quantity and quality of sleep. Components of your sleep environment are detailed below.

Medicines

Many prescription medicines can have effects that alter or decrease sleep. I encourage my patients to, if possible, control when they take their meds to minimize effects on sleep. For example, if their diuretic makes them urinate every hour for six hours after they take it, let's have them urinating while they are awake. So take this med in the morning. Other medicines may cause sedative-like effects. Take those at night. This is not exactly rocket science, but every bit helps.

A word about hypnotics, or sleep aids, prescription or otherwise: Avoid them if at all possible. While they may give you quantity of sleep, they have severely damaging effects on sleep quality. Many essentially do not let you get into the deep regenerative sleep, so you awaken not feeling refreshed, needing coffee to stay awake, then find yourself unable to fall asleep due to excessive chemical stimulation and needing something to help you sleep—and the cycle repeats.

Caffeine

Caffeine is a weak stimulant that really only pulls forward your ADP stores and energy from later in the day, which will make you more energetic now but cause a harder crash later. Caffeine does have some beneficial effects and may reduce risk of Alzheimer's. However, the most important thing to know about caffeine is its half-life of six hours. This means that 25 percent of the caffeine in your cup of coffee at 7:00 a.m. is still in your body at 7:00 p.m. And your espresso with dinner is with you all night. Liver disease can increase caffeine half-life by ten- to twentyfold. Do I drink coffee? Yes, not every day but occasionally.

Activities

The time immediately before sleep is not the time to cure cancer, solve world peace, or plan the next twenty years of your life. If you must do one or all of these things, then write the thoughts down, place your pad at your bedside, and close your eyes. Start your bedtime routine, deep breathing, and meditations. Try to meditate five minutes per day. Everyone has time for that.

Toys/Devices

The bedroom is not the place for i-Devices, TVs, earbuds, e-readers, and the like, except for what you need when you are on call. Remove these from your bedroom at least one hour before sleep. The blue light from these devices stimulates your brain and does not allow you to get ready for sleep. If you must watch TV or work on your laptop before bed, wear some blue light-blocking glasses or use the blue light-minimizing setting on your devices.

Light

If at all possible, complete blackout is best for sleeping. A study was performed where subjects had a small light placed on the back of their legs during sleep. The subjects had worse sleep quality and quantity. Black it out!

Sounds

Silence is golden, but random sleep sound machines can be useful as well. Use what works for you.

Temperature

Cooler is better. Studies show that more deep, restful sleep is facilitated by subjects not being overly warm during sleep. Cooling your room, temperature control pads, and adjusting your sleeping attire will help bring you some nice, cool sleep. I am not saying you must sleep in the nude or outside, but cooler temperatures in the bedroom facilitate better sleep.

ADJUNCTS FOR SLEEP
Your Bed

You do spend one-third to one-fourth of your life in your bed. Don't skimp on it. We finally got a new bed after fifteen years, and I have not slept better. We prefer the Tempurpedic Cloud Supreme, but try many and use what works for you. The only downside of loving your home mattress is that you become incredibly spoiled and may have trouble sleeping while traveling.

Melatonin

There is definite evidence that melatonin, for short time spans, increases sleep quantity. The sedative effect seems to wane with chronic use.

Routines

Having a set sleep routine can be difficult with the crazy, variable schedule of a physician, but on the days you are not on call and whenever possible, try to give yourself a set routine of activities that let your body and mind know it is time for sleep. This can be as simple as brushing your teeth and getting into bed, or as complex as enjoying a certain tea, wearing special PJs, reading a book, letting your dog out, and then putting on your sleep mask. Whatever works for you is best, but make it a routine.

Meditation/Deep Breathing

Clearing your mind before sleep allows you to be ready to relax and sleep. I find a very small amount of meditation before sleep puts me right to sleep. A little game I play with myself is counting the number of breaths before I fall asleep. Usually, I don't make it to ten. Sometimes it is as few as four. Yes, I can drop off like a rock. If I happen to wake up and can't get back to sleep, a few meditating breaths get me back to sleep.

Sleep Apps/Devices

Apps for tracking your sleep exist and may give you insight into progress or changes you are making in your sleep habits. Most track you by sound and motion while asleep and then interpolate sleep quality and quantity based on those parameters. Some will use heart rate and other signs to determine sleep and sleep quality. Plus, it is quite funny to hear the recordings of yourself snoring. My kids find it absolutely hilarious.

Can't Get to Sleep? Insomnia

Insomnia is an insidious sapper of energy, initiative, and your zest for life. When my burnout was pretty severe, I had significant insomnia. It absolutely compounds burnout by reducing your energy reserves for dealing with the next day's activities. Lack of falling asleep, mid-sleep cycle insomnia, and early morning awakening with lack of returning to sleep are the typical forms of insomnia. Medical conditions, caffeine intake, and the inability to turn off the squirrels running around your brain can definitely contribute to insomnia. Attack your specific problems. For me, turning off my brain is always the big problem. What I do is this: Take care of those brain-whirling tasks during the day, write them down, get them out of your brain, close that door, and then get to sleep or back to sleep.

As the importance of sleep has been recognized, a World Sleep Day has been instituted. It is held on the Friday before the spring vernal equinox and before the daylight savings time change in parts of the United States, when clocks are advanced an hour and that hour of sleep is lost until the fall. It is an annual celebration of sleep, issues related to sleep, and hopes to decrease the burden of sleep problems. Plan on celebrating next year with me! But if you miss me, I might be napping.

Sleep is critical to your life and health. Poor sleep may be a large component of your burnout. Fixing it can be extremely beneficial to you. I do always tell my patients that if any of my educational materials I give them are too dry and boring, save the reading material as an insomnia aid. It will put you right to sleep. I would advise you to do the same with this section of the book!

FITNESS

What if I could prescribe a medicine for you that would decrease your all-cause mortality by 50 percent? Decrease your risk of heart attack, stroke, cancer, and diabetes all with one miracle pill? Would you take it? Would you at least want to know what it is? OK, drum-roll, please! That miracle pill is...EXERCISE! And we are not talking about running marathons on a weekly basis or becoming the next Arnold. The amount of exercise needed to achieve these benefits is thirty minutes three to four times a week. The type of exercise is not critical, but getting greater than ninety minutes per week of exercise, with even as little effort as simply walking, reduced all-cause mortality in 46 percent in a prostate cancer study group versus controls.[63] Additionally, a recent study looking at more than 122,000 patients with an eight-plus-year average follow-up showed that as cardiorespiratory fitness (CRF) increased, all-cause mortality declined by up to 80 percent with no upper limit of benefit.[64] This study is essentially saying you can exercise yourself into great, healthy old age and reduce all your risks of death. Giant! Unbelievable! Groundbreaking!

The difficulty for physicians is always finding time to exercise. When do I have time to exercise? When I give myself permission to do it, and make it a priority. I only started to exercise regularly when I told myself that I was worth it and it was a priority. Once that decision was made, the time took care of itself. Prioritizing time for fitness has to fit within the rest of your life. Since we know that fitness will reduce your all-cause mortality, that seems like a component of your life deserving high priority. See the sidebar for suggestions for creating time in your day. Nike and I are telling you to "Just Do It." As always, do what works for you.

---

63 S. A. Kenfield, M. J. Stampfer, E. Giovannucci, and J. M. Chan, "Physical Activity and Survival after Prostate Cancer Diagnosis in the Health Professionals Follow-Up Study," *Journal of Clinical Oncology* 29, no. 6 (February 20, 2011): 726–732.

64 K. Mandsager et al., "Association of Cardiorespiratory Fitness with Long-Term Mortality among Adults Undergoing Exercise Treadmill Testing," *JAMA Network Open* 1 (October 19, 2018): e183605.

You may say, "I don't have time to exercise or do [X]." I have one suggestion, which is applicable for this entire book: *Put down your damn phone.* According to Nielsen, the average smartphone user in 2018 spent two hours and twenty-two minutes per day on their phone.[65] And I don't mean using the phone talking to patients or other medically related tasks. I am talking about time spent on nonclinically relevant tasks such as social media. Delete your social media apps. Studies also show that levels of depression are directly related to the amount of time spent on social media. Turn off notifications for all nonessential apps. Feel better, have extra time, and improve your life. Put down your damn phone. You are welcome!

NUTRITION

Too often as physicians, we eat (when possible) only to fulfill hunger or needs to continue to do our jobs, with little regard to quality, quantity, or effects on our health and life. I am absolutely not a paragon of nutritional virtue or excellence, but I do continue to learn and experiment with diet and supplements to see their benefits and effects on me. This is a continually evolving practice. Nearly every day, I feel like I learn a new fact or have a new insight as to how my nutrition affects me, my mental and physical health and my energy. Be aware of how the food, beverages, and supplements you put in your mouth affect how you think and feel, your energy, and your performance.

There are multiple different diets or ways to consume calories: Paleo, Atkins, Fast Metabolism, Zone, Mediterranean,

---

65   The Nielsen Total Audience Report, Q1 2018, Copyright © 2018 The Nielsen Company (US), LLC. All Rights Reserved.

DASH, Flexitarian, Intermittent Fasting. All seem to have their own unique properties and ways to help people control and/or lose weight. I am a giant advocate of what works for you. Recently, I have learned about the Blue Zones and the nutrition associated with those colorful zones. The Blue Zones are the areas of the world where the populace routinely lives very healthy, active lives into their eighties, nineties, and even more than one hundred years old. Staying active and connected to a life purpose, your community, a Higher Power, and eating a largely plant-based diet are key characteristics of the lives of the inhabitants of the Blue Zones. These seem to be a diet and lifestyle that works for me. Try and use what works for you.

Try to avoid things that will make you feel worse. Sometimes you may not know how bad a particular food or product is making you feel until you eliminate it. It is an iterative process and will take time. Eliminating one item at a time will provide you with the maximum feedback.

TOXINS

Our modern society produces significant benefits for us, but like it or not, the by-products of modern living are the toxins that we are exposed to on a regular basis. Anything we can do to minimize exposure to harmful compounds in our environment will aid in your physical recovery from burnout. BPA, nonstick coatings, aluminum foil, environmental estrogens, and a host of chemicals that seem to end up in our groundwater can accumulate in you with unknown effects. The fewer of those unknown chemicals that end up in your body, the better.

The Environmental Work Group (EWG) Healthy Living App lists and rates more than 120,000 food and personal care products. It is an excellent resource for assessing the products you use every day, what their toxic rating is, and what are some minimally toxic alternatives.

SUPPLEMENTS/VITAMINS

Nearly everyone has a favorite supplement, herb, or root that seems to work wonders for them. I like to use anything that has some positive real research behind it, seems useful, not harmful, and that I can tolerate. Multivitamins in small doses seem to have beneficial effects. However, my stomach is like a delicate desert flower and I cannot tolerate multivitamins. I like and use a resveratrol supplement as the scientific evidence is large and compelling, I tolerate it, and it seems to improve my mood and energy. I use a nicotinamide supplement for better cellular energy production and utilization, and it improves my sleep and workout recovery.

An excellent resource in the supplement arena is *The Supplement Handbook: A Trusted Expert's Guide to What Works & What's Worthless for More Than 100 Conditions* by Dr. Mark Moyad (Rodale Books, 2014). Mark is a tireless investigator and advocate of evidence-based use of supplements. He has put out quite a useful compendium of information about exactly what the title says: *What works and what's worthless*. He is a friend and great patient advocate. Trust what he has to say.

The bottom line for your physical health and nutrition is to try something, anything, and I can almost guarantee you will feel better, increase your energy reserves, and combat burnout. Increasing your health, fitness, and nutrition will directly and effectively decrease your burnout. I encourage you to keep reading, learning, experimenting, sleeping, and eating! Begin the urban renewal project today! Get back on a first-name basis with Gym! "But how do I pay for all of this?" you may ask. The next chapter will enlighten you.

CHAPTER 12 TAKEAWAYS

- Your body is your support system for your life.
- Treat your medical conditions, Doctor!
- Maximize the controllable, beneficial components of your health.
- Exercise without limits. It does a body good.
- Food is fuel. Use the premium grade.
- Minimize the toxins in your environment.
- Supplement with care.
- *Put down your damn phone.* You're welcome!

CHAPTER 13

Your Financial Wall

"Anyone who lives within their means suffers from a lack of imagination."

— OSCAR WILDE

TRAPPED?

Finances and money can also be a primary driver for burnout. You can feel trapped in your current situation. You may not like the work, or the call, or the EMR, but if you need to make X dollars to cover your expenses and the only way you know how to make X is what you are currently doing. You are trapped, at least financially, for the time being. This does not mean you cannot change your income or expenses, save to make a change or a host of other avenues we will explore. But you may feel and be slightly trapped now financially. This financially trapped feeling also increases any burnout you may be having as well. Let's use your imagination to change your parameters and open the trap to get you out.

I am not suggesting you expand your imagination and spending but open your mind to new ways to think about all things financial. This may be the most impactful wall, as most people and physicians tend to expand their expenditures to match their means. I am acquainted with someone who lives paycheck to paycheck on more than $1 million per year.

There are many informative websites and resources for investing, financial information, financial planning, robo-financial planning, and even so-called FIRE—Financial Independence/Retire Early. I am not going to try to regurgitate or re-create all that admirable content. Investing is certainly one avenue to pursue to give you more freedom and independence. Once your investment income exceeds your expenses, you can reduce your reliance on direct work and W-2 income or leave medicine entirely.

As physicians, we have jobs that typically provide a good income. But those jobs also come with golden handcuffs chaining you to a golden treadmill that keeps you running and trapped. It is very difficult to imagine stepping off or changing the settings on the treadmill, or finding a completely different "exercise" to pursue for fear of loss of income, prestige, respect, privilege, or ego. The list of reasons to keep running is nearly endless. A very wise man, John Corman, my co-chief resident at UCLA, said to me, "Jeff, we have the best job in the world twelve hours a day. It's the work during the other twelve hours a day that can kill you." So from a financial standpoint, how do you get loose from—or better yet, avoid—the golden handcuffs and treadmill and find time to do the hot yoga/mountain biking/CrossFit plan?

PRIORITIES

Determine your answers to these questions:

- What are your financial desires?
- What are your goals?
- What are your motivations?
- Are you trying to beat someone, to make more money than [fill in the blank] your father, brother, friend, neighbor?
- Do you always win, no matter what the game, even one you really don't want to win and shouldn't be playing in the first place?
- Are you making a bad compromise like, "If I do this (horrible) job for five years, then I can do what I really want to do"?
- Are you letting money determine your behavior? "The money is so good that I am willing to sell my soul to [fill in the blank] the devil, hospital, group..."
- Are you just hanging on until things get better? "I will make partner in two years, then my call will only be every third night and I'll make 10 percent more. Yippee!"

What I am proposing is that you begin to think and consider expanding your universe and mind about your current financial situation. I want you to open your mind about the nearly endless options for income and ways to change your expenses.

Let's talk about the revenue side of the equation first.

INCOME

I recently attended an excellent conference in Chicago hosted by SEAK, Inc., which highlighted nonclinical careers for physicians, such as performing expert witness work, chart and disability review, writing, speaking, consulting, investing, and teaching. First, know that these are all employment opportunities that any physician is immediately qualified to perform. Second, these relatively simple opportunities for using your clinical skills in nonclinical ways do appreciate the value that seven or more years of medical education and decades of experience are worth. Third, most of these opportunities have very low costs or no cost for you to initiate.

Consider what the going rates are for some of these opportunities:

- **Expert witness work:** $250–$1,500 per hour.
- **Chart and disability case review:** $100–$200 per hour.
- **Writing:** Pay varies by job and type but can range from a small stipend for an article to thousands or more for a book.
- **Speaking:** Some physician speakers command $20,000–$30,000 per engagement.
- **Consulting:** Either an hourly rate of $250–$500 per hour or by the job from $5,000 to nearly unlimited, depending on scope and results. Working as a paid consultant for large firms like McKinsey can start at $200,000 per year for full-time employment.
- **Investing:** Venture capital firms, biotech startups, medical equipment companies, and more all need medical expertise. These arrangements are individual by the job but could lead to a full-time position as well.

Let's do the math for a second: Say you are doing chart review and are paid $200 per hour. This is work that can be done on your own time and at your own pace. If you did ten hours per week of this, that is an extra $100,000 per year. If you do expert witness work at $500 per hour, take only two to four cases per year and that might amount to four hours per week, that is an extra $100,000 per year. I know a physician who alternates between working in practice for six weeks and expert witness work for six weeks and makes over $1 million a year for his expert witness work.

What I want you to consider is what an extra $100,000 per year allows you to do. Would that let you go to a part-time status? Could you reduce or eliminate your call or night-time duties? Can you accelerate your investing or reduce debt to get to financial freedom sooner? Extra income from small-time commitments greatly expands your options, reduces stress, can actually be fun and intellectually stimulating, and most importantly, frees you from the trapped feeling of your financial wall.

What if you love what you currently do and do not wish to add hours of other work to your week? You should explore the possibilities of monetizing what you currently do for free. For example, how many committees and boards do you serve on for other money-making organizations (your hospital, health system, practice, etc.) and you receive no pay for your time and expertise? Ask for pay for your board time and expertise. Ask for medical directorship pay for leading hospital improvement efforts. Ask for pay for being on call. Explore gain-sharing arrangements for improving healthcare performance and saving money in patient care areas.

There are endless opportunities for receiving value personally for the value you bring to others. As physicians, we are not trained to think this way. But we do bring incredible value, not only to our patients but to the organizations in which and for which we work. It is right, appropriate, fair, and time to receive that value. But you have to believe you are worth it and ask to receive that value. All organizations love to get the milk for free without paying for the cow. Stop being milked. This will also reduce your burnout, as you are valued for your expertise. I am only scratching the surface of what is possible.

Your income opportunities are nearly endless, the world is your oyster, and you merely need to lift your head up and look around to see what is available to you. And instead of making $40 per work RVU, you can actually be paid for your worth and expertise to a virtually unlimited degree. For you, the sky is literally the limit for income.

EXPENSES

The other side of the financial wall/burnout equation is your expenses. Doctors classically have large incomes and equally large expenses. I am sure part of this is due to the nearly endless delayed gratification that we undergo during our training and the perverse societal perception that doctors are rich and should show off their riches. I have never understood this, but it seems to be a real expectation by society.

But regardless of your income, it is always possible to increase expenses to an equal amount. Expenses are really what your priorities are. Your priorities set your spending habits. If it is important to you to wear a certain type of clothes, drive a certain car, and live in a specific neighborhood or house, that is all predicated on your own priorities. If you want to change your expenses, change your priorities.

Get out your financial wall paperwork. On the left, write down what your priorities are and what they cost you. On the right, write down what you want your priorities to be and potentially what that would cost or save you. In the middle, write down the steps from where you want to be, starting from where you are. Again, start from the end and work backward if that is easier to visualize. Write down what you actually spend your money on. To get the most accurate picture of your spending, for one month, tabulate the large categories of your spending. Your bank statement, credit card statement, and bills will account for the majority of your spending. This exercise will point out to you what your spending priorities are. Does your spending match your actual priorities? There may be large expenditures that have nothing to do with your priorities. Those may be expenses that can be eliminated, simplifying your life and decreasing your need to generate income to cover them.

Do a separate financial wall worksheet for your income. Include current income sources and streams on the left. On the right, add potential income sources and total value of each one. Chunk out the steps from left to right to get from where you are to where you want to be. And just for fun and clarity, put totals to each column for both income and expenses. This will give you a very powerful illustration of what your priorities are costing you, how you can change and improve them, and what a life-changing impact some simple attitudinal adjustments and asking for value in exchange for the value you create for others will do for your life.

Finance, income, revenue, and expenses are not sexy, fun, or exciting, but they do determine a very important part of your life box construction. They are important causes and cures for your burnout. They are the parameters that define what is possible for you. Be very deliberate about how you construct your financial life, what your priorities are, and how you are compensated for the value you bring to others. Once you have completed the reconstruction of your financial wall, your burnout will decline dramatically. It only takes a bit of imagination, as Oscar Wilde would ask you to employ. Now that your finances are in order, ask yourself if your spiritual house is also in order.

CHAPTER 13 TAKEAWAYS

- Income does not equal freedom. We have to keep running to make more.
- Do your goals and priorities match your income?
- Are you making bad compromises?
- You have nearly endless opportunities to create value for yourself based on your education and training.
- Small investments of your time can equal large residual income, which can create freedom and opportunities in your life.
- Ask for compensation for value you create already.
- Match your expenses to your priorities, not your income.
- Complete the steps to get from where you are to where you want to be.

CHAPTER 14

═══

Your Spiritual Wall

"Faith is taking the first step even when you don't see the whole staircase."

—MARTIN LUTHER KING JR.

A man was sitting on his roof, flood waters rising around his home. A neighbor rowed by in a canoe. He called out, "Do you want a lift?" The man on the house replied that his faith would provide for him. A rescue crew in a boat motored up to the home, and again, the man demurred, citing that faith would provide. Finally, with the water near the top of the roof, a large raft with other flood victims floated by. The man did not accept their offer for a ride, again declaring his faith. The man drowned. Arriving at the entrance to the promised land, the man asked the gatekeeper why his faith had not provided for him. The gatekeeper replied, "I sent three boats!"

Having faith is important. Acting on your faith is critical as well. Taking the first step, as Dr. King advises, treats your burnout. Do you act on your faith? What is faith? How do you know that the sun will come up tomorrow? How do you know when you are in love? When a miracle occurs in your life, how did that occur? The common element in all these is faith, a belief in the unseen, a Higher Power or energy. Faith is nearly a universal thought system in the world with hundreds of religions based on it.

There is an increasing amount of evidence that we humans are, indeed, life forms of energy and power that exist now in physical form. Thoughts and bodily processes are transmitted by electrochemical impulses, which like all electrical impulses, also emit magnetic waves. And these waves interact with each other and the universe. What kind of energy waves are you generating? Positive? Peaceful? How are you perceived by others? Granted, these are energetically very weak waves, but both the electrical and magnetic impulses can be detected with current technology. We do not have technology with the granularity to fully sense and interpret these waves and their effect, if any, on the surrounding environment or vice versa. In fact, *Science* magazine's 125th anniversary issue classified the question of the biological basis of consciousness as one of the top twenty-five remaining scientific questions.[66] We may not have a Super-Duper Mind-Reading Detector (SDMRD)—yet. But lacking that absolute empirical scientific evidence, what we do have is faith, or a belief in a Higher Power. Good old-fashioned faith and belief sustains a large majority of the world's population on a day-to-day basis.

So how is your faith? And by that, I do not mean I am questioning or judging if, what kind, or how much faith or religion you may practice. I am asking about whatever level and energy you use for your faith. What I mean is, do

---

66 https://www.sciencemag.org/site/feature/misc/webfeat/125th/

you allow a belief in a Higher Power to enrich your life? Do you allow personal, familial, work, and larger miracles a place in your life? Do you have happy accidents?

I am not rooting for any home team from a religion standpoint, but I do think it is critical to allow for and accept that there can be a locus of control, power, energy, luck, love, and beauty outside of yourself. There is a certain freeing aspect to the consideration that a Higher Power exists and has a place in your life. Accepting, or at least acknowledging, this concept is important for several reasons.

First, it takes some of the pressure off you. As doctors, we somehow think we have the God complex, that we are our own Higher Power and have absolute control over all things medical. And subsequently, by extension, we doctors control the rest of the known universe. Unbelievably, 100 percent of what happens in your life may not be under your complete control. The stress and pressure "to be God" as a physician can be overwhelming and add to your burnout. Let the Higher Power take the wheel, especially when something quite random, good, bad, or otherwise seems to just occur in your life. "Wow, I just saw my high school best friend, unplanned, in Morocco." "I am completely astonished at that patient's stage IV cancer's spontaneous remission." "I found my car keys!" Once you allow for some faith-based serendipity, you can release your own personal belief that you control and are responsible for all events happening in the world. Not only is the belief that we are completely in control extremely weighty, tiresome, and stressful, but it is a tad arrogant as well. Yep, we are not gods. Stop acting and believing as if you are one. Your life, body, energy, and stress level will thank you.

Burnout declines when the pressure and stress you place on yourself declines. OK, sermon over.

Second, faith can give you a framework for continuing your efforts when all other evidence is to the contrary. There are definitely dark times in all of our lives. There are times when we doubt ourselves and our plans. Faith in what you believe to be the course of action will keep you going when pretty much everyone else has quit or told you to quit.

Third, faith can be incredibly comforting and give peace. When I have had a particularly stressful or bad day, a few minutes of meditation, release, and what I can only call interacting with my Higher Power is reassuring, relaxing, comforting, and energizing. Doing this allows me to refocus on what is important and have some perspective on the events of the day. I am nothing if not a bit of a "hot reactor" to situations, so this exercise has a calming influence on me as well.

How can you increase faith in your life? Am I asking you to attend religious services eight hours a day, donate all your time and money to organizations of your choosing, or simply become a person of the cloth? No, I am not, but those are all options open to you. If there is one thing I want you to learn from this book, it is that you have essentially infinite options regarding how you construct and live your life. What I am asking you is to be open to making changes in your life that will be beneficial to you. Life is not necessarily what happens to us, but how we respond to it. Consider the role of faith in your response.

ACTIONS TO INCREASE FAITH

MEDITATE

Do this at least five to thirty minutes per day. Find a quiet place. Close your eyes and only focus on your breathing, in and out. That's it. Simple, I know, but it is a practice that seems to be passing the test of time, like for more than 3,500 years. Meditation will allow you to more directly connect with your faith. Do it. It is said if you don't have time to meditate five minutes per day, you should start meditating an hour a day.

LOOK FOR SMALL MIRACLES

"Look at that, a parking spot just appeared where I needed one to be." "Hey, my case is starting thirty minutes early, so I can get home to see my daughter's concert." Recognize small miraculous occurrences and be grateful to the Higher Power for the little blessing that just popped into your life.

BELIEVE IN SOMEONE ELSE

Put your faith to work, and put it in someone else's hands. Let someone else help you. And don't sneak around double-checking their work. Just believe!

GIVE PEOPLE THE BENEFIT OF THE DOUBT

Sometimes, having faith means believing that someone else may have a different way to accomplish a task or not necessarily do it exactly the way you would have. Give others some leeway in their process, and they will surprise you, usually pleasantly.

BELIEVE IN SOMETHING

Believe in a cause or a task strongly. Put that belief out there in the universe so the Higher Power knows you are working on it. Work toward it, and almost always, help in some form will come running toward you. Try it.

ACCEPT THAT A HIGHER POWER IS AT WORK

Hey, more than six billion people can't all be wrong, can they?[67]

This is not an exhaustive list, just mine. Use these as you see fit. Add your own. Have faith that you will determine what works best for you. Get off the roof, on the boat, and participate in your own spiritual life. Take the first step on the stairs. Believe that you can recover from your burnout. You are now ready to interact with the world. Let's go be social!

CHAPTER 14 TAKEAWAYS

- Faith is an important component of your box and life.
- Faith asks for belief in energy within and outside of yourself.
- Allow faith to relieve your own personal God complex, give confidence to continue action, and instill peace.
- Meditate, allow a place for faith in your life, and act on your faith.

---

67   David B. Barrett et al., *World Christian Encyclopedia: A Comparative Survey of Churches and Religions in the Modern World* (New York: Oxford University Press, 2001).

CHAPTER 15

Your Social Wall

"Never miss a party...good for the nerves—like celery."
—F. SCOTT FITZGERALD

As physicians, the nature of our work practically forces us to be social with our patients, colleagues, partners, and coworkers. It is a bit of a daily work party, as you meet all sorts of interesting characters who become your patients—sans celery, of course. (There are certain specialties in medicine with little to no direct social contact with the patients. We picked out the people in our medical school class who would be well suited for those particular specialties, primarily for their lack of current social skills or preference for the inanimate over the living.)

THE SIDES OF YOUR SOCIAL WALL

When I think and talk about the social wall of your box, there are two sides to that particular wall as they relate to burnout. One is positive and the other can be considered negative. The negative side of your social wall consists of the social interactions, energy loss and drain that being sociable, or not, can bring. This side can increase burnout. Let's proceed down the Debbie Downer path for just a minute.

As a physician, there is a social contract you engage in as part of your job. You are asked to be social enough to assess a patient's health, history, physical exam, and studies and appropriately treat the patient, regardless of their response. The negative aspects of this social contract that you have may include being pleasant in the face of a drunk patient screaming obscenities at you in the middle of the night while you are trying to help them. Or having to be very patient with patients who are trying your patience, such as spending thirty minutes debunking the fifty pages of internet search information they have on herbal treatments for aggressive, advanced cancer.

Sometimes, at the end of a particularly draining day or a long call night, the last thing you want to do is to be social and your reservoir of patience is low. I can guarantee you from personal experience, your well of patience will run dry. You will lose the battle between the mental and social filters in your brain and your tongue. You will say or do something inadvisable, and it never works out well for you. There will be a hurt, angry patient at the other end of that interaction, a guilty, remorseful physician, and if you are lucky, a complaint to Google or Yelp, your practice administrator, a hospital administrator, or the medical board.

Here is some absolutely free advice: If you feel yourself losing your cool, excuse yourself from the situation, get help from a friend or partner, and either recollect yourself with a new, calmer attitude, or have someone else take care of that patient. Not every doctor or patient will react to an interaction in the same way. We all have our hot-button issues, and some people just have the right mojo to push those buttons. It is OK to say no to a situation that you know will end badly. And sometimes, time away from negative social interactions will allow you to recharge and be ready for another day.

One technique I use when faced with a difficult patient is putting myself in their shoes. Having empathy for patients is critical to our profession, but it is one of the first casualties of burnout. This loss of empathy is described as depersonalization. If I was just told that I had cancer or needed surgery, or I did not understand what was happening, how would I feel? That gives me a fresh perspective on why they might be aggressive, argumentative, or abusive to me or my staff. They are scared and don't know how to react. My job is to help them through that. Perspective and empathy aid in your role as trusted advisor.

So to reiterate: When your reserve is low and you are about to say or do something that you will undoubtedly regret, put yourself in their shoes, or disengage gracefully, regroup, and either have a new plan and attitude or pass that patient off to someone else.

The sad face side of your social wall exists. You cannot ignore it, but you can work with it. The positive side of your social wall is remarkably beneficial, empowering, uplifting, and actually lifesaving.

There are numerous studies that demonstrate the positive effects of social interaction, including the Blue Zone work of Daniel Buettner. These effects include and are not limited to longer life, lower blood pressure, lower incidence of heart attack and stroke, and lower incidence of depression.

To be completely honest, my favorite part of my job is getting to know the cool, funny idiosyncrasies and details of my patients while helping them with whatever problem is plaguing them. I have patients who are world-class photographers. I have patients who have helped countries set up their financial systems. I have professional sports Hall of Fame patients and Olympic Gold medalists. There are many patients to whom I say, "I want to be you when I grow up." In addition to whatever their medical problems may be, they are people with lives, stories, emotions, and talents. They are complex, interesting, and have an amazing capability to enrich and improve your life while you are improving theirs. This is the positive social side of our interactions.

In addition to your social interactions with patients, open your mind to the concept that one of your key social interactions is your human connections with your colleagues, partners, and coworkers.

The work we do as physicians can be stressful, energy draining, frightening, and extremely sad at times. Only another person who works in the field can understand what we go through. This understanding is your bridge from them to you when you need support and the way you support others in their time of need. I cannot tell you how many times I have had a particularly bad day or experience, and after I tell a partner or colleague about it:

1. I feel immediately heard and feel better.
2. I get a new perspective and new ideas on how to deal with a situation.
3. I feel gratitude toward my listener.

4. I get help, from a practical standpoint, with whatever was going on.

Sometimes this means a partner will see a patient or do a case or surgery for me while I deal with whatever else is happening. Sometimes this means I will just go home. Lean on your support system when you need to and give yourself that permission to access it. No more trying to be the Super Doctor! And be the support system for others when they are in need. It is absolutely a two-way street. The giving and receiving of support are vital components of your burnout recovery.

You must realize and then embrace the truth that humans are social creatures. We cannot, as much as we try, remove millions of years of genetic encoding that makes us crave and need social interactions. These are the ties that bind, enrich, and empower our lives. Please do not discount or downplay them.

Finally, you are not alone. Nothing makes burnout burn more brightly than the incorrect view that you are alone, no one has ever gone through something like you are experiencing, and no one can help you. The feelings of solitude and isolation can definitely lead you into a downward spiral.

The best remedy for feeling less alone is to not be alone. Interact actively with your family. Join a support group. Join a club of something of interest to you. Take opportunities to invite others to join you for a coffee, a meal, or an event. Increase your social interactions. You may be somewhat of an introvert. This may be hard. But one small move in a positive direction will make an unbelievably large improvement in your outlook. You will feel less stress, more connection, and now have a support system to engage with when burnout rears its ugly head again. You just have to try. And if your attempts at socializing do not seem to be working, if your feelings of isolation are not improving, if you cannot find your own sounding board, seeing a therapist is also an excellent option. The isolation of burnout decreases with more social interaction, either in formal or informal settings.

One exercise I can recommend is to try to add positive social interactions to your day, every day. Let's say you are going for a coffee. As you order, look the person directly in the eye, note their eye color, smile, give them your order, give them a sincere compliment (I like your outfit, thanks for being so cheerful, thanks for taking my order so quickly, cool piercing, nice ink...), and accept any comment they have in return gracefully. Most often, the other person is so surprised and pleased to have been given a sincere greeting and compliment that they will beam and smile. And both of you feel better and have great starts to your respective days. I do this exercise multiple times a day with my patients, and it is an awesome way to instantly generate a positive social connection. I have a 95 percent success rate of getting a smile out of the other person.

If you feel there are other aspects of your social wall that need to be addressed (no one likes me, I eat alone, I am the only one who has ever gone through this, etc.), use the three-step process outlined previously in chapter 9 of defining where you are and what the problem is, where you want to be, and work forward or backward on it. Put a definite success assessment end point for each step. You define what success looks like. Give yourself a deadline for every step, so then you know when you have achieved it and the goal will have some built-in urgency for you to complete.

Your social wall is an important component of your box. The negative side can be improved, and the positive side is your friend and savior. The connections we feel and have with others help us live a complete life. Please don't neglect all the wonderful interactions you can have in your world while enriching someone else's. Have some celery, improve your nerves, and be social!

Your box is now complete, with the exception of something to cover the top. Let's examine your ceiling.

CHAPTER 15 TAKEAWAYS

- Medicine requires social interaction with patients, and those can be positive or negative.
- Controlling your reactions when faced with scared, offensive, or difficult patients takes patience, empathy, trying on their shoes, and maybe another physician's perspective.
- Find the interesting, positive social interactions with your patients.
- Develop, lean on, and contribute to your social network of colleagues.
- You are not alone!
- Be social and practice creating social connections.

CHAPTER 16

Your Ceiling

*"When you reach for the stars, you may not quite get one,
but you won't come up with a handful of mud either."*

—LEO BURNETT

What if you built a house without a roof? You would always be getting wet. The last component of your box is the lid or the ceiling. What does the ceiling represent? If the floor is your past and the walls are the present, then the ceiling is your future, or what you believe to be possible for yourself. With respect to burnout, the ceiling represents hope and what is possible for you when your burnout is improved. The ceiling can also represent the limits you and your burnout have placed on you. "I can't do that. I am too tired/pissed/trapped/frustrated..." You pick the adjective to describe how burnout limits you and your ceiling.

However, if you reach for the stars, as Mr. Burnett suggests, you will not get mud, and you will most likely blow through your ceiling while reaching for a star. The ceiling is the limits you have either consciously or unconsciously put on yourself about everything in your life: what you do, how you do it, why you do what you do, how much you make, where you live, with whom you live, and your maximum potential.

The vast majority of people do not plan to fail, plan to be burned out, or plan to have a less-than-satisfying life. People fail to plan or to examine their own ceiling. Without planning for the future, you cannot ever achieve the vision or even see your ceiling. How do you construct your ceiling? First, set personal expectations and goals as high as you can possibly imagine. Think, dream, and mentally construct the ideal life for yourself. That is your ceiling. Then do the work on your walls to support your ceiling.

Let me give you an example. I was thinking about writing this book. "I am not a writer," I thought to myself. "What do I have to say?" "How do you even go about writing or publishing a book?" "I could never write and publish a book." Those are some pretty severe limiting self-beliefs and self-doubts. My ceiling was so low that I was bumping my head on it constantly. Then, while listening to a podcast, I learned about an intriguing way to publish a book either by simply being interviewed as a subject matter expert and having the book written, or writing the book yourself and having the company shepherd you through the publishing process.

The publishing company is amazing, and I really like the feel, vibe, and philosophy of the company and the people with whom I interacted, including the founder. This is not a free service and the cost is significant. The cost was enough to stop me in my tracks: "I guess the universe just doesn't want me to write this book."

Wait. What? Nothing was stopping me. Except me. I was finally able to see that my personal and financial limiting self-beliefs were the ones stopping me, not the universe, and I had to call BS on myself. I sat and wrote down ten different ways I could afford the price. I had enough confidence in myself and what I learned over the past twenty years about myself, burnout, recovery, and expanding my thinking that I then wrote and published this book. Writing the book itself was cathartic for me, but that really was the easy part. Deciding to write the book and not stopping until that happened were the hard parts. I had broken through my low ceiling.

Do not let your limiting beliefs determine your life. Blow through them. Set really giant, high, seemingly unbelievable goals and then do the work to get there. Set a BHAG! What is a BHAG? A big, hairy, audacious goal! This term was coined by Jim Collins and Jerry Porras in their 1994 book, *Built to Last: Successful Habits of Visionary Companies*. It is meant to inspire strategic, empathic goal setting for long (ten to thirty years) time frames while motivating teamwork and efforts with smaller BHAGs set along the way. Define your BHAG and get moving on it!

A word about timing and action: For heaven's sake, *take action* and do something now! Otherwise, in a week, month, or year from now, you will be as burned out as ever or even worse. You'll also be one week, month, or year older and most likely not be wiser and possibly sadder. Do it now!

Let's set a goal and define your action plan. Get something to write with.

1. What would be the most audacious incredible goal you could accomplish in the next year?
2. Why is that goal important to you?
3. What resources do you need to accomplish that goal?

For example, let's say your goal is double the number of patients you can see in the next year. That would be an impressive feat.

Why is that goal important to you? Perhaps you live and work in an underserved area or work in an in-demand specialty with limited access, and patients are not doing as well as they could due to poor access to you.

What resources do you need to accomplish seeing twice as many patients? There are still only twenty-four hours in a day and only one of you. I am a huge fan of doing only what you can do. If your role is as a surgeon, your specific tasks that only you can do are assessing the patients and performing the operations. Delegate or outsource the other tasks you usually do during the day. How do we leverage your time and efforts? Hire a scribe or two to take away the EMR time sink. Hire physician's assistants or nurse practitioners to do the pre- and postoperative care and rounding. Streamline office processes to allow more patient volume. Use multiple exam and operating rooms to maximize your efficiency. Do not take on more work for yourself. Using a few of these suggestions will radically increase your efficiency, patient volume, and happiness without burning you out, and accomplish your BHAG: doubling your patient volume!

At this point, we have blown up, torn down, and reconstructed the floors, walls, and ceiling of your box. It has been a monumental task even thinking about, analyzing, assessing, and reconstituting your entire life, piece by piece. Congratulations! Mr. Burnett would be proud of you for reaching for your star. But you must know that your new box comes with change, actions, and fear. Those sometimes can be disconcerting.

CHAPTER 16 TAKEAWAYS

- Your ceiling represents the limits you place on yourself.
- Set your goals as high as you can imagine.
- Take action toward your new goals. Nothing will change if you do not.

CHAPTER 17

—————

What a Nice, New Box You Have!

"The beginning is the most important part of the work."

— PLATO

Whew! You made it through the entire box. Congratulations! You have started on your new beginning. And yes, I know, my box is more of a hexahedron. It was not intended to be casket-like in its shape, but you get the analogy.

You have considered your agreements. You have defined your "why." You are forming new habits. You have refinished your floor by moving from where you are to where you want to be in steps of your choosing. You have questioned your work environment. Your mind has been expanded to new dimensions. You have a fitness and nutrition plan. Your money activity matches your priorities. Faith is your copilot. You have become the cruise director of your social life. And your ceiling is covered with the stars you are reaching for. Congratulations!

It is a process, and you are, in fact, assessing your entire life, deconstructing it, reconstructing it, and planning the steps to get you there. Fricking overwhelming! Good job. I only expect you to make the progress you are ready to make. But I would ask you one thing: Take one step on any of the actions of any surface of your box. Just one. Your new you will thank you!

The inertia of remaining at rest is great. Do not rest too much. Do not fail to START. Why go through all of this and do all the work to START to make a change and then quit? There are absolutely no points awarded for getting to here and stopping.

As you go through this process, you will feel confused, tired, frustrated, and "lost" perhaps.

That is normal. That sensation of disorientation is one part of your identity changing, and you do not quite yet know how to reidentify who you are. This is called liminality, which is defined as a transitional period where you may not feel you have a defined social role, or that role is changing and you have confusion regarding your identity.

In medicine, doctors almost always think and act as if we know or are expected to know everything. During this life and career reassessment period, you will definitely not know everything. Hence, you will be sensing that liminality, that disorienting feeling of loss or change of your current identity, such as doctor, board member, department chair, chief of staff, managing partner of your group, trapped, burned out, or suicidal. You are transitioning to a new identity: open, hopeful, aware of possibilities, at peace, entertaining multiple options and career possibilities, and being a new kind of doctor. Trust me. Liminality is your friend in this transition. Just know that it can and will occur and roll with it. Instead of struggling against it, understand that this is a natural part of change and not a signal to retreat back to the old, unsuccessful ways and the old, familiar box of your previous life.

Great job on building your new box/life! You have completed the most important part: the beginning. Plato and I are proud of you. If your personal attention deficit disorder does not allow you to possibly work through the comprehensive box reconstruction we just detailed, then the next section with the QuickStart guide may be just what the doctor ordered.

CHAPTER 17 TAKEAWAYS

- Start!
- You have a new life and new box!
- This process will feel disorienting, scary, and unfamiliar. That's OK!
- Do not let liminality stop you from creating your new life.

CHAPTER 18

The QuickStart Guide

If you are like most physicians, your patience for anything is small. And if you are digesting information, you want to do it in the most efficient, fastest way possible. You never read the manual for any device. You just start using it or, at most, read the QuickStart guide. If you read nothing else in this book, this QuickStart guide can give you a rudimentary outline about how to quickly get a start on your burnout recovery. Going through the full wall-by-wall process is the preferable, best, and most effective way to pursue your recovery, but I put this here because I know a lot of doctors!

FIVE STEPS TO DO *TODAY* TO REDUCE BURNOUT

Burnout is an insidious, career- and potentially life-threatening disease. It did not occur overnight and will not necessarily get better overnight. However, there are steps you can take today to immediately reduce your burn-out TODAY!

1. Acknowledge
2. Accept
3. Assess
4. Align
5. Act

ACKNOWLEDGE

The first step of diagnosing a problem is acknowledging one exists, as in all good twelve-step programs and most medical issues. Be aware that you have a problem.

ACCEPT

Everybody likes to think they are on top of everything and we have it all under control. Well, let's just say that you probably would not be reading this if you didn't have a little smidgen of a hint of a thought that you may be burned out or not so on top of things. Take off the cape, Superman or Superwoman. Life is tough and demanding, especially as a physician or healthcare provider. It will be OK. Just accept that you possibly cannot do it all, and you may need help. We physicians are the worst ever at asking for help. Ask already!

ASSESS

There are four components here.

One: What makes your blood boil? That is about the shortest line between you and burnout. I mean what causes serious frustration and may not be necessarily in your control, and you may or may not have already attempted to fix said craziness without success. But still, there is no resolution or improvement and the problem continues.

Two: What are your priorities? No, really, what are they? Not God, country, and brussels sprouts, or whatever you say your priorities are. What you spend time, energy, money, and focus on are your priorities. List them now. I'll wait. OK, got them written down? Which ones are needs, and which ones are wants? You need sleep, food, exercise. Just about everything else is negotiable and adjustable. Let's focus on the wants. These are the ones you can alter and reduce most easily. For example, I wanted to be the highest producing partner for my lifestyle, ego, whatever. But the toll it is taking on me, my life, my health, and my family is ridiculous and excessive. Refocus on your actual priorities. Refocus on your needs. Your family needs you. Your patients need you to be at your best when you are with them. You have to make the choices. Back up the ego bus and get focused on your real priorities.

Three: What is under your control? Let's break this view of life into two parts: things in your control and things out of your control.

IN YOUR CONTROL	OUT OF YOUR CONTROL
Your response to everything in your life	The world, accidents, traffic, bad bagels
Your schedule	Lateness by others
Anticipating outcomes	Unforeseen complications
Reacting badly to unplanned outcomes	My EMR is not great
Time allocation	Patient factors
When you leave for work in the morning	
Getting help to run your EMR efficiently	

Be creative here. Think of different ways to attack the items within your control, which really is just about everything. Life happens, and 99.5 percent of what governs the quality of my life, your life, everyone's lives is our reaction to what happens. Acknowledge that and own it. Say it one hundred times: "My reaction governs my quality of life. My reaction governs my quality of life. My reaction governs my quality of life..." Ninety-seven more to go. Not kidding. Do it!

So think, plan, anticipate, and course correct when the inevitable unplanned events occur.

Four: Imagine a perfect day. How does that look? How does it feel? What do you do? What steps would it take to make that perfect day a reality? Money is no object in this thought experiment. This feels and looks a bit different than your current life, right? Go back and think of what things on your wish list that you can incorporate right now. Rearrange your schedule and take a day off a week. I did it after only eighteen years. I am a slooooow learner, as you can tell. That was a lifesaver and a game changer for me.

ALIGN

Take your actual priorities and align your time, energy, money, and focus with those priorities and make a burn-out recovery to-do list!

ACT

Find the most doable step and do that right now. Put down your laptop/tablet/phone/smart watch or whatever you are reading this on, and do it right now. You cannot come back to this until you do. Alternatively, you can give yourself an ironclad deadline for completion of the task, which triples your chances at success.

OK. You did it, right? Good job! Cross it off your burnout recovery to-do list. Tomorrow, you can start on the rest of the list. Or if you are feeling super-motivated and energetic, do more now. The beauty of taking action is that you are back in control!

That wasn't so bad, time consuming, or awful, was it? Congrats, you just got the quick and dirty secrets to curing burnout and having a more focused, meaningful, less burned-out life. You are most certainly welcome!

REMEMBER THE FIVE AS!

OK, QuickStart guide over! Let's get back to our regularly scheduled user manual.

CHAPTER 18 TAKEAWAYS

- Do the five "A" steps above if you cannot rebuild your whole box today.
- Action is the most important of the five As.
- I know if you are doing the five As, your attention deficit disorder does not really allow you to read more here.

CHAPTER 19

What I Do

"The cosmos doesn't owe you a thing. But it does reward thoughtful, ethical, and determined effort."

—SCOTT PERRY

A personal section of this book about things I do that have been helpful should have a disclaimer: None of what works for me is meant to be a line-by-line prescription for you. Try some things. Give it some "thoughtful, ethical, and determined effort" to treat your burnout. Determine what works for you. This section also includes some insight into myself. Throughout this book, I have attempted to be true to myself, you, the reader, and burnout. This is my voice. If and when we meet—and I hope we do someday—you will find that speaking with me is like reading my book. It is an exercise in congruence, authenticity, and alignment.

I finally realized how energy draining it was for me to "be the doctor" like some omniscient deity or at least play that part at all times. I have never identified myself as a doctor, except when I am in an exam room or the operating room. And even then, if you were my patient (and I hope you do not need to see me in that capacity), this is what you would hear: me assessing and explaining things in my voice and most likely using humor to relieve any anxiety you have. I know physicians who are always in the "doctor/expert" role, socially, financially, when exercising—whenever. It is exhausting for me just to witness it in someone else. If that is your true personality, then own it. If not, it is unbelievably draining being the expert, or pretending to be, at everything at all times, especially when you may not be. And the psychic penalty of "being wrong" personally and professionally seems high for you. It is only a job, profession, career. It is not you or your being. Get off your high horse. Yes, what we do is serious. Yes, we deal with the life, care, and death of others, but realize the effects this career can have on your life. A little distance and perspective can do wonders for your mental health and happiness while decreasing your burnout. An appreciation of other medical career options and the opportunity to escape the imprisonment that the clinical practice of medicine can be affords you hope about your future. You are not trapped. You feel better about yourself just because you know you're not trapped in your role or your job and you're working toward something else.

As I continue through my burnout recovery process, I am more open to other options. I am less stressed, less boxed-in, less married to outcomes, and more invested in the process. As I consider other career options, I am less angry and frustrated, less focused on nonsignificant work metrics, less argumentative, and more able to see a broader perspective. I am also taller and more handsome! No, not really. But I am improved on a number of fronts. I know, being more open-minded does seem to be a panacea. It is difficult to explain it until you experience it. But looking back to my pre-burnout treatment days, the changes both inside and outside of my life are significant. Ask my wife and family!

MY PROCESS

It drives me crazy (Holden Caulfield-esque) when an entire informational or self-help book goes by and the author never talks about what they do or what works for them. It is probably because the author has not tried, done, used, or been successful with any of his described techniques. Not me! I have kissed the toads and tried many processes, supplements, books, theories, dictums. I have read libraries of self-help books, done yoga (which I think is awesome!), and traveled across the country for various conferences. Below are what I have found to be useful to me.

I am going to tell you what I tell my kidney stone patients: I am giving you a number of techniques and ideas. Pick one or two that you like and think sound good to you, and try those and do those! If, after a sincere effort, which is whatever constitutes an effort for you, what you are trying is not working, then try something else. This is not an exact science. Everyone is different, and what works for me may be completely unhelpful for you.

But I think that the searching process for techniques or tips that work for you is a useful exercise as well. Habit science says it takes approximately thirty days to instill a new habit, so give yourself a month to see if some of your new habits have sunk in and are useful.

WORK LESS/WORK MORE EFFICIENTLY

No tombstone has ever been inscribed with the epitaph, "I wish I had worked more and harder." As physicians, we are wedded to the unbelievable work ethic that was drilled into our collective heads prior to and during medical school and residency. Unless we are working at full speed and literally flying down the hallway with our hair on fire, we are clearly not working hard enough. We have a joke that physicians are happy about five minutes per year when our level of busyness is just right. Otherwise, we are absolutely too busy and getting killed, or not nearly busy enough and just sitting around. At least, that is what we think.

Let's be completely clear: Some of this work mania is of your own creation. The box you have constructed may now have you trapped. It is difficult to approach solutions from within your place of constraints. Consider that working less may certainly mean less income. You may need to expand your box, develop other streams of income, or reduce your expenses, expectations, and lifestyle burn rate.

At this point, really, I want to bring this to a hard stop. Throw your life in "park." The crux of all of this is whether you value yourself enough and consider yourself worthy enough to fix this problem. You have to think highly enough of yourself and love yourself enough to want to make changes to improve your life. Value yourself enough to stop, look around, and realize the degree of your happiness or unhappiness and the degree of control that you have over that situation. I finally decided to value myself enough to begin change. I valued myself enough to give myself permission and time to care for myself.

And let me be completely clear: The critical aha moment that allowed me to even consider working less was severing the link between my ego and self-esteem, as we explored previously. I revalued myself enough at a new, slightly lower level of productivity. The mental paradigm shift was acknowledging that I was still a good doctor and productive partner without being number one! But the paradigm shift was the critical step. The end result was working less and working more efficiently, which decreased my burnout and opened my life for more life!

It took me more than a year of working less than full time, at least on a days-per-week basis, to finally arrive at a point where I could actually disengage my mind enough from medicine and reengage in other parts of my life. I started to take Fridays off. Of course, I changed my schedule on the other days of the week to accommodate and add back in the appointment slots I had deleted on Fridays, but the ability to physically not be in the office or the operating room freed my mind up for a significant chunk of consecutive free time not thinking medical thoughts. I also enforced the Fridays-off protocol and did not add on "just one case." That never worked. It turned into an all-day work fest, and I ended up feeling burned out and resentful because I had worked all day. So Friday off means Friday off.

I started reading nonmedical books again. I started listening to and buying music again. I started seeing giant increases in the number of ideas I just spontaneously had for improvements in my practice, business, and my life. I exercised much more regularly. My family told me I stopped looking and being mad all the time. And, believe me, they told me beforehand how bad I was getting. This was completely fair, appropriate, and left no room for less-than-massive change.

Also, working less was critical to gaining some perspective and allowed space to write this book. It allowed me the time, energy, and direction to expand back into other areas of interest. I also gave myself permission to explore something, really anything, outside of medicine.

I have always very much enjoyed teaching, and I am now reentering that sphere. I believe that I have something worthwhile to give by educating other physicians and healthcare providers about how to change and control their lives and take back their careers while they still have a chance. I have an interest in business, the economics of medicine, and ways to improve the patient experience.

To those ends, I cultivated some relationships at the University of Denver. I was a volunteer judge for student presentations on healthcare at the college of business there. Subsequent to that, I suggested that there might be some practical lectures that students would benefit from outside of the standard business fare and consisting of life lessons and pearls accumulated through years of experience both in and out of medicine.

I'm sure you're familiar with the maxim that if you show interest about something, you will get promoted to do something about it. I am now an occasional visiting lecturer in the Daniels College of Business at the University of Denver, presenting to first- and second-year students in a business communication class about the psychology of business, money, and success. The opportunity to lecture these students has probably been more therapeutic for me than educational for them. But I do hope they have learned something from me.

I am writing this book because I always thought I "had a book in me" and this was a way to share my trials, tribulations, thoughts, learning, and benefits with other physicians and the world. In writing circles, this is known as the Hero's Journey. And through this process, I have rekindled my joy for teaching and recaptured my zest for life.

TRY SOMETHING NEW, AND PLAN ON FAILING

As my family will tell you, I'm something of a nut for gadgets. I have an all-electric battery-powered snowblower. I very much enjoy cooking with my smoker. Recently, I read a newspaper article about air frying and subsequently bought an air fryer and air fryer cookbook. This was a fairly inexpensive purchase, and we have had a lot of fun as a family trying out new recipes and cooking—or burning, according to my family—different types of food.

Five or ten years ago, I would've never had the patience to purchase another device for me to then maintain, use, or tolerate any sort of less-than-perfect result, as my self-constructed box and my life did not allow time for fun, experimentation, or failure. So this has been a fun, happy experiment and a good use of time.

EXERCISE

I do cardio exercise two times per week for thirty to forty-five minutes and weights/resistance training with P90X two to three times per week. I do yoga two to three times per week.

If I could do only one exercise, it would be yoga. It is cardio, resistance training, stretching, and relaxation all at the same time. I think it keeps the muscles and joints from ossifying further, and it is good for the mind.

MEDITATION

The scientific benefits of meditation are well known. I use two types of meditative breathing regularly. Part A: You can do this anywhere at any time. Every day, take ten slow, deep, full breaths in and out, eyes open or closed. Try it driving (preferably driving with eyes open) or whenever two or three times per day.

Part B is incredible. For five to twenty minutes per day, simply sit in a comfortable quiet position, and focus only on your breathing. In and out. That's it. If you get distracted, like the little puppy that I am inside, simply refocus on your breathing. You may want to visualize something while meditating, such as light entering your limbs and exiting the top of your head. You may want to chant a mantra in tune with your breathing, such as "Love, Abundance, Gratitude."

What has been the most uplifting has been using this meditation time to give myself a period while meditating of unabashed good feelings about myself. I consciously stop all the self-doubt, self-flagellation, and worry and allow myself to feel an upwelling of positive feelings about who I am, my abilities, my contributions, and my life. Try something and see what works for you. I have experienced significant and spontaneous happiness while doing this. That is a new experience for me. Amazing creativity and clarity also follow these meditation sessions for me.

SAUNA

I use a dry, infrared sauna heated to 120–130 degrees for ten to twenty minutes a day, if possible, or three to five times per week. The health benefits are well documented (lower blood pressure, lower stress, remove toxins), but it is very relaxing as well.

NUTRITION

I eat vegetarian the majority of the time. I have a Shakeology shake for breakfast. Subjectively, I think it has improved my mood and energy. It is filling, has micro- and macronutrients and is probably the healthiest food I put in my body all day, other than my wife's yummy vegetarian dinners. I have a salad and fruit for lunch every day.

SUPPLEMENTS

Resveratrol. As of November 1, 2019, there have been 12,371 scientific papers written about various aspects of resveratrol, which is a plant-derived polyphenol with potential or actual benefits for cardiovascular disease, obesity, diabetes, Alzheimer's disease, and cancer. Most supplements have fewer than ten papers written about them and their effectiveness, and some have none at all. I take it daily.

Niagen (nicotinamide riboside). Nicotinamide adenine dinucleotide, or NAD, is used by all cells for energy metabolism. With aging, NAD production declines in our bodies. Supplementing with NAD precursors, such as nicotinamide riboside (NR), increases the available material for energy production for your cells in your body. It has been shown to protect users from cardiovascular disease and may have positive post-exercise muscle recovery effects. Most importantly, it helps me sleep.

SLEEP

I used to be a "sleep when I am dead" believer. Not now. I try to get at least seven to eight hours per night. I do my meditation exercise to drop off. I almost never can make it to ten meditative breaths before I am asleep. I turn off all electronic devices at my bedside or put them elsewhere, except when I am on call, and minimize use for one to two hours before bedtime. I use Swanwick blue-light-blocker glasses if it is absolutely necessary to use electronic screens within thirty to sixty minutes before bed. We have a TEMPUR-Cloud Supreme mattress. This is the most unbelievable mattress on which I have ever slept. I fall asleep nearly immediately. The downside is that I have gotten incredibly "sleep spoiled" and now have some trouble sleeping elsewhere. Sleepers beware! For those of you with excess body heat, cooling pads can also be very effective. We use one called OOLER. My wife swears by it for increased, more restful sleep.

LEARNING

Learning is an aspect of life that is critical to being fulfilled, happy, engaged, and truthfully, less burned out or even burn-free. For me, it always shows the promise and path to a different, better future. I am a big fan of telling my patients that I know I do not know everything. Anything I can learn is helpful if it increases satisfaction, peace, hope, vision, and my care and engagement with them as well. As we say in the medical field, every day is a school day. If you are not learning, then you are already starting to stagnate.

Lifelong learning is something we have drilled into ourselves from a medical standpoint with continuing medical education (CME), meetings, journal clubs, clinical clubs, pathology conferences, and the like. These are all important and necessary to stay current from a medical knowledge standpoint.

Medical learning is mentally stimulating, but sometimes it feels like another job. We all follow and adhere to these commitments, and they are usually required for maintaining board certification. I do my home CME as audio downloads and listen when I am exercising on the elliptical machine, so I get exercise and education at the same time.

When I say learning, I am also talking about feeding your brain nonmedical new ideas, thoughts, and fun! I am a big fan of technology to maximize this learning time. I download podcasts to my iPad to listen on my commute, which is about twenty-five minutes each way. I love my Airpods to listen to books, podcasts, or talks when open audio would be rude or disruptive to my environment. I used my phone to dictate ideas and parts of this book to later incorporate and integrate. I use the Otter app, which records and simultaneously transcribes your dictation very accurately. I love it! I use Audible to read me books when I am exercising or driving. I use Blinkist to quickly review books that I "have been meaning to read" for six to twelve months.

I hired a research assistant on a per-job basis through the freelancing website Upwork to do some of the heavy lifting when it comes to research specifically for this book. Personally, trying to do research always leads me down a rabbit hole after which, two hours later, I have nothing to show. Thanks, Ursula, for saving me from my own research black hole! Learning about anything and getting your brain out of medical thinking for a significant portion of the time you are outside of the office, operating room, or hospital is necessary and will keep you sane.

DIVERSIONS

I pursue a number of diversions now, up from nearly zero several years ago. I love to cook and make some mean ribs, chicken burritos, and chili! I took a pencil drawing class at our Fine Arts Center. It was mentally exhausting and exhilarating at the same time. I was surprised by how much I enjoyed it.

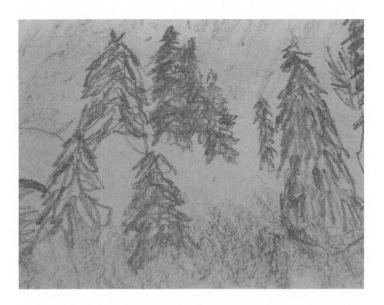

I am a sucker for Tom Clancy and Jason Bourne-like novels. I have a slowly growing collection of single malt whiskeys. I have a large crazy sock collection. I am part of a poker group that has met monthly for the last twelve years.

WHAT I DO SUMMARY

The preceding suggestions are just part of an amazing laundry list of things to do and try. I actually do 75 percent or more of this list every day. Explore your own interests and pursue them. Work less so you have time to do that, and give yourself permission to pursue them as well. All of what I do has made for a quantum reduction in my burnout. I now have a much higher self-awareness of my burnout triggers. I immediately employ measures to change, improve, and counteract those triggers. I have learned how to diagnose, treat, and recover myself from burnout.

WHAT HAS NOT WORKED FOR ME

Let's also talk about what has not worked for me. Over-the-counter medicines or occasional alcohol use provided only temporary improvements in sleep, with return to poor sleep cycles and sleep hygiene. I have not used any other recreational or pharmacologic prescriptive drugs to help with recovery or sleep. This seemed like a dangerous path to go down as pharmacologic methods for sleep are not really in tune with our bodily functions and ultimately work against you.

From a financial standpoint, I am a lifelong nonbudgeter, at least as far as writing one down. I am horrible at that. What I do is prioritize my needs, then wants, and set up automatic spending for those. I also have not balanced my checkbook in fifteen years. But I do closely track our accounts. This is what seems to work for me.

In retrospect, it is enlightening to consider my mental state "BB," "B," and "PB"—Before Burnout, Burnout, and Post-Burnout. BB, I was relatively happy-go-lucky, unconcerned about current or future problems, and able to let things roll off my back. During B, my emotional reserve did not allow me to easily bounce back from problems.

I perseverated on minor issues, and there seemed to be a baseline level of frustration and discontent that colored everything I did. "Why should I help fix that problem at the hospital? It will never change." "I am too tired and pissed off to enjoy this time with my wife and family." During B, there was a qualitative change in how I perceived everything. All things required too much effort. There was never enjoyment from any activity. Whatever I did was just another job, even when I was camping with my family or having a nice dinner with my wife.

Now that I am PB, I do not consider myself "cured." Burnout does not lend itself to a once-and-done fix. But I see myself regaining perspective, peace, and having an awareness of the old burnout triggers, identifying them and short-circuiting their effects on me. It is almost humorous when something that previously would send me into a downward spiral for days or weeks is now something that I notice, realize how I had reacted to it DB, and use my new paradigms for progressing toward a healthier response.

It's not always perfect, and I am not always successful in my responses, but at least I have the awareness to be present and choose from an array of positive actions. Claim your reward for your efforts. As previously stated, burnout treatment works best when both personal and institutional changes are affected. It is time to look at your institution.

CHAPTER 19 TAKEAWAYS

- Be yourself, not THE DOCTOR.
- Do what works for you.
- Work less. Work more efficiently. Pretty simple. Hard to do.
- You are worth the effort!
- Reconstruct your life to allow more life for you.
- Reconnect with what you love and brings meaning to you.
- Fail! It is a wonderful stress reliever.
- Care for yourself: exercise, eat well, sleep, learn, explore.

PART IV

Institutional and System Fixes of Burnout

CHAPTER 20

Our Healthcare System

A Giant Box?

"The hospital will not love you back."

—VAGABOND MD

NEPTUNE CALLING?

There are times I do feel the hospital is not loving me back. Recently, we were informed by our hospital system that (congratulations) our urology group was now on call for several more rural hospitals, some up to three hours away from our location. There was no discussion. This was not a request.

Did the planet of Neptune need urology call coverage as well? Can we please take that on? Or was Neptune already included in this newest mandate? The burden of this additional call coverage by itself is not large but yet another responsibility heaped on the current mountain of work.

This story illustrates how systemic drivers of burnout can be significant as well. To effect changes in our systems, we must better understand how those systems are created and function. In this chapter, I want to give you the background and tools to understand, cooperate, change, and improve your system, all with the goal of reducing your burnout.

Just as we personally may have a box of our own construction in which we live and work, the healthcare system in which we participate, work, and use has its own boxlike elements. Granted, we have 1 million percent more control over our personal box, but we should at least understand and appreciate the parameters of the healthcare system box. Once you understand the structure, it becomes more possible to make changes to it.

The base level of construction, or the floor, are the rules and regulations with which we all comply. These are handed down by the federal and state governments and our respective state medical boards. On top of those, we have the walls of requirements from our educational institutions and our specialty-specific governing boards for board certification.

We need a place to work, so healthcare institutions and hospitals grant us the "privilege" of using their facilities for diagnostic, inpatient, and surgical services, which is another wall. For that privilege, the economic benefit generated for a healthcare system, per provider, is not small. Data shows that depending on specialty, a single physician can generate between $1 million to $5 million annually in revenue for a healthcare system.

Ultimately, it would be nice to be paid for the services we provide. Thus, we apply to participate in private and public insurance panels so patients can use their insurance coverage to see us, which is another wall of the systemic box.

Additionally, the tax code creates its own wall and is written in such a way to incentivize most healthcare systems to not show a profit to maintain their not-for-profit status. All monies are then reinvested back in the healthcare system. Have you ever noticed how many construction cranes there are at a hospital?

This leads to interesting situations where if there is extra money in the system, it must be spent. It cannot be used to lower prices or decrease costs. This seemingly does not incentivize more cost-effective care. But, again, this is a result of the tax and regulatory requirements imposed on the system.

Systemic regulation is necessary to ensure appropriately trained physicians are caring for patients. That is a given. But the other part of the equation is the requirement of certain duties to maintain full licensure as a practicing physician. For example, we are required to maintain hospital privileges to stay on insurance panels. This makes perfect sense as payers want to ensure that their covered lives have facilities and doctors to access care. But if I have hospital privileges (required by insurance), then the healthcare system requires me to be on call to cover their facility. For the majority of my career, and for most specialties and facilities, this was an unpaid requirement. As the burden of call coverage increased, we did finally advocate for ourselves and now receive slightly more than some states' minimum hourly wage for covering the hospitals in my area 24/7/365.

Another wall is the governmental electronic medical record reporting requirements. To date, EMR requirements have not been shown to improve care, but they still take me hundreds of hours per year to complete and, for my practice, nearly two full-time equivalent personnel to maintain. The ceiling of our system box is the maximum capacity for work and patient care. The rules and requirements of healthcare facilities are essentially immutable. Those parts of our system box do not seem to be under our potential control. So what can we do to improve our situation?

As research shows, physician-only burnout solutions have some beneficial effect. However, combined solutions with both personal and institutional changes show the most positive, durable effects. According to a 2018 survey, the top five factors physicians report would reduce their burnout are increased compensation to avoid financial stress (56 percent), more manageable work schedule (31 percent), decreased government regulations (27 percent), more reasonable patient loads (24 percent), and increased control/autonomy (23 percent).[68]

I agree wholeheartedly with all of those recommendations, or what I would call a wish list. Any and all of those would be helpful. The real questions are how to achieve those results. In addition to personal investment and change, institutional changes are necessary and corequisites.

There is now at least institutional awareness of burnout and the part healthcare systems may play in its increase. I implore hospitals, healthcare systems, and institutions

---

68   IQVIA, *Physician Office Usage of Electronic Health Records Software: Market Insights Report* (Irvine, CA: IQVIA, May 2018).

to stop giving lip service to burnout. It's not enough to provide watercolor painting classes, resiliency classes, and doctor appreciation days or hours. Healthcare institutions need to stop requiring more and more from their physicians.

I am not saying that we physicians do not appreciate those efforts. But those are top-down, management-style approaches to addressing the results of systemic problems. They do not address the problems. Can we effectively treat a rupturing aortic aneurysm with Band-Aids and blood transfusions? No, we need to treat the source of the problem. From an institutional level, we need to replace the rupturing aorta with a new graft. Can we replace or repair the parts of our systems that engineer harm to our physicians?

Let me propose a path forward with some ground rules. I encourage you to work with your system or employer using these ground rules to effectively move forward and reduce your burnout.

GROUND RULES FOR EFFECTIVE PHYSICIAN/ HEALTHCARE SYSTEM CHANGE

1. In order to fix systemic problems, all facets of the system, good and bad, inside and out, physician-related and not, will need to be examined.
2. This will take time, money, resources, flexibility, and willingness to change by all.
3. This will be a cooperative effort. The system will contribute resources and open-mindedness. Physicians will contribute open-mindedness, effort, ideas, and feedback.

4. There will be no billboarding or trumpeting of results for individual system gain.
5. All useful results, both positive and negative, will be freely shared with other systems and, if appropriate, published in peer-reviewed journals.
6. Credit and acknowledgment will go to the creators, but the knowledge and benefit will accrue to all.

Can we all play nice with those ground rules?

Let's use the following as your playbook for interacting with your hospital and system partners.

COMMUNICATE

Without information and interaction, no system can diagnose and solve its own problems. The fastest method to obtain this information is to have active communication with its users. There is a giant reservoir of experience, information, and ideas for improvements in a healthcare system in its physicians. Historically, this has been untapped. Make use of this resource by communication.

ASK

A question will never be answered if it is never asked. Ask, include, dig, query, discern, uncover—use smoke signals or send carrier pigeons if you have to—and get the information set necessary to define what is right and what is wrong with your organization. I do not recall ever being asked what I think is wrong with the system.

PARTNER

Collaborate with your doctors. Now that you are communicating and asking your doctors, find out what is driving their burnout, what ideas they have for progress, and what their pain points are. Share data. Give feedback. Interact. Doctors as a group are a relatively smart bunch. Capitalize and incentivize physicians to participate in their own system redesign and personal recovery. If gains and improvements occur from the work, improvements, and efforts of physicians, share those benefits! Once it becomes obvious that we are reimagining medical care for the benefit of all, including physicians, I believe physician help will come out of the woodwork.

There is sometimes an undercurrent of competition and/or distrust between physicians and healthcare systems. There is fear that when one side learns something, they may use it to their advantage. The ground rules should eliminate those concerns.

Healthcare systems need to prove their commitment to partnering with physicians. Trust, honesty, and integrity are earned over time by following through on collaborative plans and actions. Physicians need to trust administrators as well.

ENGAGE

A very large-scale Gallup poll showed high-performing businesses have a statistically significantly higher rate of what they call employee engagement.[69] Employee

69   Gallup Press, New York, NY 10019, Library of Congress Control Number: 2017957145 ISBN: 978-1-59562-208-2, 2017, Copyright © 2017 Gallup, Inc.

engagement is defined as workers feeling they are performing meaningful, significant work in a culture of personal improvement.

Almost by default, you would think that physicians feel they are performing meaningful work as they try to positively impact the health and well-being of patients. And I would say personally I do strive to impact each patient positively and I derive much satisfaction from those interactions. However, that feeling of meaningful work can be washed away by menial tasks doctors are asked to complete every day.

Additionally, the engagement criteria of a culture of personal improvement may exist, but physicians are not given time to access those resources. The demands of the job, productivity metrics, and the extreme regulatory and malpractice environment may decrease the chance to access personal improvement. Some areas, such as tort reform and reexamination of the utility and success of previous governmental regulation, are necessary but well outside the scope of this book.

EMPATHY

Physicians perceive we are considered just a cog in the machine, a number, or a commodity. We are perceived by some healthcare systems or employers as eminently replaceable. Because all doctors are exactly the same as far as experience, knowledge, empathy, energy, work ethic, and talents, right? No, not really. Caring about me, as an individual and a physician, and valuing the contributions I make in time, energy, effort, risk, and literally, blood is all

I ask. That is really all any of us ask. Recognize me as an individual, what I contribute, and what I sacrifice. Listen and act on my concerns and drivers of burnout. If there are EMR system issues, communications challenges, or negative outcomes in the hospital, what avenues can be explored for resolving these problems?

One solution could be a hospital floor, or operating room "facilitator" or "fixer." This person would roam care areas, ask questions, and assess needs for physicians or the care units, communicate understanding and empathy with their frustration, and quickly act on solutions. This person would be a rover in the hospital, going to where needs or problems seem to be most acute.

Just as there are patient representatives for patient needs and concerns, this person would be a system representative or ombudsman available to serve physicians, nurses, or anyone else with a problem in need of a solution. And in the unlikely circumstance where there are no current, urgent problems or needs, that rover can solicit feedback from patients, staff, and physicians about what is going right and record that as well.

Any or all of the above will definitely fix systemic problems and reduce burnout!

CONSTRUCT

We can build a new system around physicians with one primary goal: Make physician wellness the top priority. Organize, plan, and rearrange behavior to achieve just one goal: physician wellness.

WHY?

1. We, as a system, are in dire need of positive change and run the risk of losing an entire generation of physicians and other providers to despair, burnout, early retirement, and death, either from stress-induced illness or suicide.
2. The current abuse-based training and dysfunctional healthcare systems have reached the end of their lives.
3. We lose four hundred physicians—the equivalent of one medical school—to suicide each year.
4. Physicians are the engine and the decision-making core of the healthcare machine. If the engine is broken, missing, or dead, the system grinds to a complete halt.
5. The current system with its growing, endless demands and more finite resources is not sustainable.
6. There will be unbelievable improvements in patient care, physician productivity, and sustainability of healthcare as an integral part of our society with a physician-wellness-focused system.
7. It is the right thing to do.

I am not blaming hospitals or institutions. But those organizations that employ more than 50 percent of the physicians in this country are in an outsized position to affect change. Strictly from an economic standpoint, those administrators and systems who grasp this concept and employ a positive, active, evolving culture centered on physician wellness will have a competitive advantage. Can you imagine the positive public relations that would come from being known as "the best hospital/healthcare system in America for doctors and nurses to work for"? I would seriously consider moving and reducing my salary requirements to work at the best hospital in America for physicians.

HOW?

If we have set physician wellness as a keystone behavior and defining priority to ourselves, our institutions, and our healthcare systems, now what?

Once a priority is set, organizing behavior around that is relatively straightforward to achieve that goal. What are chief drivers of physician burnout and poor physician wellness?

1. Personal "box" factors as delineated previously.
2. On-call responsibilities, time commitments, interruptions of regularly scheduled care, life, and sleep.
3. Time/productivity benchmarks not linked to patient or physician satisfaction.
4. Processes ill-designed for maximal ease of use and productivity.
5. Electronic medical records—all aspects—including but not limited to user interface, lack of personalization and humanity, interoperability, productivity drain, and so forth.
6. Recognition of extra effort for all the intangibles: time, caring, phone calls, attending funerals of patients with whom physicians had significant relationships, dedication, effort, and going that "extra mile."

WHAT?

Action Steps. These are best derived and decided on at a local level. What works in Mobile, Alabama, may not work at all in Minot, North Dakota.

1. Personal box reconstruction as detailed previously.

2. Expand physician call coverage options. Add/employ dedicated "call teams." Allow local/regional triage services to assess and coordinate care more appropriately and directly. (As of now, there is incredible duplication of services at nearly every hospital in a local or regional area.)

3. Link productivity to patient, physician, and healthcare system satisfaction, safety, and population healthcare metrics, not merely to patient throughput in service lines.

4. Reengineer processes to maximize physician efficiency. Engage with physicians for highest value strategies.

5. Decrease or eliminate physician interaction needed to complete non-physician tasks. Make or let physicians do what only physicians can do: facilitate seeing patients, doing surgery, making patient care decisions. Remove impediments to care (e.g., EMR data entry, prior authorizations process, pharmacy medicine change requests).

6. Add personnel and/or technology as necessary to create an efficient utilization of EMRs (scribes, data entry, voice recognition software, etc.), or require requests for proposals (RFPs) from EMR vendors to include usability, safety, and interoperability benchmarks.

7. Encourage and incentivize better overall health in a global view for the patient. Reward provider efforts supporting communication, empathy, access, health metrics, *and* volume but not *only* volume as in our current system.

8. From a physician mental health standpoint, develop a dual-track physician health program where administrative, legal, or substance abuse referrals are handled through one branch with current regulations and

oversight, and another path that would be exclusively for mental health referrals, including self-referrals, without need for a sentinel event or bad outcome. This would be an open, transparent process with no possibility for licensure action. This would radically decrease the fear, stigma, and concern about utilizing this great resource. As PHPs are state-level organizations, physicians should contact the PHP in their own state and ask about current structure, what options there are for treatment, and the privacy of that treatment. A larger effort would be to restructure PHPs in this two-track plan to allow all the care for all medical professionals who need care.

I know this is a new, giant, impressive, ambitious list to attack. Pick one! Pick something! Start!

Meanwhile, after returning from Neptune to take care of a patient, we can see how systemic box construction exists and we have opportunities to make changes, on Earth and in your neighborhood system as well. Working together, maybe we can get our hospitals to love us back.

Systemic change is a critical component to fixing the entire "burnout ecosystem." Making physician wellness a central goal is an excellent avenue to reform our healthcare system from the inside out, while improving and potentially ending physician burnout. Doing so will take energy, cooperation, caring, and focus. This has been an amazing journey. Thank you for taking it with me. Let's put a bow on your box!

CHAPTER 20 TAKEAWAYS

- Your healthcare system is a box.
- Set ground rules with your healthcare system for productive analysis and change.
- Communicate. Ask. Partner. Engage. Empathize. Construct.
- Systemic improvement is the right thing to do from patient, physician, system, social, economic, risk, and care viewpoints.
- Design your system and your life around physician wellness, including mental health.

CHAPTER 21

Conclusions

Tying It All Together

*"I leave this life with no regrets. It was a wonderful life—
full and complete with the great loves and great endeavors
that make it worth living. I am sad to leave, but **I leave
with the knowledge that I lived the life that I intended.**"
(Emphasis mine)*

—CHARLES KRAUTHAMMER, MEDICAL DOCTOR,
PRESIDENTIAL SPEECHWRITER, NATIONALLY
SYNDICATED COLUMNIST, QUADRIPLEGIC, JUNE
8, 2018. PASSED AWAY ON JUNE 21, 2018.

Let's move you toward a life of your own intention by treating your burnout and bringing your new "you" into being.

I did get a new keyboard, and it rests happily on my desk. I have kept the old keyboard to remind me of how this journey started, how far I have come, and how lucky I am that that was the only thing seriously broken.

Throughout this book, we have explored the journey that led us to, through, and past burnout to recovery. We have seen that burnout is real, damaging, potentially life-threatening, and treatable. Burnout has significant mental health effects, including depression and suicide, but there is help! It's increasing and does not seem to have an obvious solitary source, but we can point to potential causes—like EMRs—for improvement. Burnout can cause patient safety issues and is expensive. It is a worldwide phenomenon. In order to reduce, control, and treat burnout, it takes personal and systemic changes. There is a transition period from where you are to where you want and need to be. Be ready for that change and transition. Define the agreements that frame your box and your motivations. Create new agreements with yourself and others. Explore your box.

Find and define your floor, walls, and ceiling. Assess those surfaces. Build yourself a new box of parameters of your choosing, not ones foisted on you by others or by accident. Take action! Partner with your hospital systems to champion physician wellness as a centerpiece of every decision. Live your life on purpose, on your purpose, by design and intention. Let's fix your box and the system. Get started! You know why, where, and how!

Acknowledgments

Writing this book has been a journey, not unlike recovering from burnout. I have been aided along that journey by many people. I want to first thank my mother and father, Shirley and Don Moody, for their unwavering support, insight, and roles as personal cheering section.

My family was incredibly understanding of the early mornings, nights, and weekends of me tapping away at the keyboard. They were so supportive during my recovery from burnout and as I revealed some of my innermost thoughts and fears while writing this book. Sarah, Rachel, and Will, thank you for being one of the most important parts of my life.

My wife, Cheryl, was my first reviewer and gave me the confidence that I was on the right track and had actually "invented" something, as I promised her so many years ago. I am so lucky to have your love, insight, and guidance every day. Thank you!

The team at Scribe Media, from my initial contact, Rikki Jump, to my ever-patient and continually encouraging editor, Hal Clifford, to founder Tucker Max, who crystallized why I was writing this book, have been critical to taking an idea I had and turning it into a real, substantive, useful book. I am changed because of your effect on my life. I have no words to express the depth of my gratitude except two: thank you!

I am indebted to the Scribe Guided Author Facebook Group for providing encouragement, support, and guidance on some deep issues.

To all of you who gave me invaluable feedback on early versions of this book, you made me a better writer and the book better for your input and commentary. Specifically, I must thank Gillian McDonald, MD; Randal Schultz, JD, CPA; Jason Spears, DO; Di Thompson, MD; Brad Dresher, MD; John Corman, MD; David Penson, MD; Kolleen Dougherty, MD; Joan Burns; Alyson Motcheck, RN; Lori Ouellette, RN; Allan Roth, CFP, CPA, MBA; and Amie Sharp, MA, MFA.

My "other doctors," Mindy Graskamp, PhD, and Kimberley Johnson, PhD, provided invaluable personal and professional perspectives, as well as being familial supporters. Thank you!

My extended family—David Marcus, Rita Marcus, David Roston, and Leslie and Kyle Fitzpatrick—gave cogent input and reminded me constantly of the important things in life: family and love.

Professional colleagues Stephie Gregory from Ferring Pharmaceuticals and Lauren Beckner at Boston Scientific provided real-world validation of what I was writing about and gave practical suggestions. Thank you!

John Clarke, without whom I would have never been paid for my work as a doctor, has always been a friend, peerless mentor, and guide. Thank you for improving my book and my life!

To my partners, Buzz Walsh, MD, Henry Rosevear, MD, Gary Bong, MD and John Mancini, MD, I thank you for keeping me sane, letting me vent, watching my back, and making our practice the best place for me to be a doctor. Thank you to my "work mom," our practice manager, Stephenie Mishkofski, and the staff at Pikes Peak Urology for putting up with me for twenty years. I hope we have left you better for our partnership.

I could never have climbed out of the research cavern of my own creation without Ursula Murphy, my Upwork researcher extraordinaire and spoken edit listener! Thank you for saving and enriching this book with your expertise and informational reinforcement.

I am grateful to my medical colleagues for their honesty, compassion, caring, drive, and resilience. You prove to me every day that you are special, worthy, and deserve a life full of challenge, joy, and balance.

Finally, I want to thank my patients for the honor and privilege of caring for you. I am a better person for you allowing me to be a part of your lives. Thank you!

About the Author

DR. JEFF MOODY is a board-certified, UCLA-trained, practicing urologist with over twenty years of experience. During that time, he's survived at least six electronic medical record transitions, the Affordable Care Act, and practice consolidation. He's also served on numerous local, state, and national healthcare organizations. Dr. Moody knows the warning signs and challenges of burnout personally, having lived through the diagnosis, treatment, and recovery. In addition to this book, Dr. Moody supports his colleagues by sponsoring a monthly Physician Burnout Support Group. For more information or to connect with Dr. Moody, visit JeffMoodyMD.com.

Made in the USA
Las Vegas, NV
11 July 2024

92173666R00135